NUTRITION AND DIETETICS

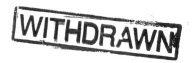

Campion Integrated Studies Series

NUTRITION AND DIETETICS

A Practical Guide to Normal
and Therapeutic Nutrition

F. Pender
N. van Kaathoven
N. van Mierlo

Campion Press

British Library Cataloguing in Publication Data

Pender, Frederic
Nutrition and Dietetics:Practical Guide
to Normal and Therapeutic Nutrition in
Clinical Practice. – (Campion Integrated
Studies)
I. Title II. Series
613.2

ISBN 1-873732-09-0

© 1994
Campion Press Limited
384 Lanark Road
Edinburgh, EH13 0LX

Cover design:
Artisan Graphics, Edinburgh

Typesetting:
ParaText, Ratho

Typeset in Bookman 10/12

Printed and bound by
Alden Press, Oxford

Preface

Module 1: Food, behaviour and practices

Chapter 1 addresses the issues and concepts of the non-nutritional factors governing food intake and includes social and psychological circumstances and religion. **Chapter 2** considers the roles of both the dietitian and the nurse and the interaction necessary for the provision, monitoring and evaluation of both basic and more specialised nutrition. It takes the reader from encouraging a patient to eat a proper diet through to the routine observations and measurements that allow the nurse to monitor a patient's progress. The module concludes with an account of factors affecting a patient's ability to eat.

Module 2: Nutrition and health

Chapter 1 introduces the concepts of basic nutrition and includes descriptions of accepted definitions and criteria of under- and over-nutrition. It highlights factors influencing the development of altered nutritional status. **Chapter 2** explores the basis of a healthy diet and describes basic informational tools to assist ideal food selection such as the food guide. The concept of nutrient quantity and quality is addressed together with aspects of food quality, safety and use of additives. Food labelling is studied. The principles of general nutrition are fully explained. **Chapter 3** looks more specifically at individual nutrients. A systematic study of significant nutrients addresses the sources, functions, requirements and consumption levels of macronutrients (protein, fat, carbohydrate, energy) and micronutrients (vitamins and minerals). **Chapter 4** introduces the context of nutrition in relation to specific groups of the populations. Nutrition of the infant, toddler, schoolchild, adolescent, in pregnancy, breastfeeding and the elderly are considered. In particular, focus is placed on nutrient requirements and food selection. **Chapter 5** considers the effect of advertising on food selection and choice by the media, packaging and image of the food.

Module 3: Nutrition and health problems of today

Chapter 1 introduces the reader to the common diseases in society in part attributed to faulty diet and/or lifestyle (coronary artery disease, cancer, bowel disease). General and specific recommendations are made for reducing the risk of developing such diseases. **Chapter 2** considers the various types of eating disorders and in particular emphasises the social context in which they arise. The aetiology, prevalence and treatment are explored of both anorexia nervosa and bulimia nervosa together with the major characteristics and psychological problems facing the victims. **Chapter 3** emphasises the sources of food poisoning and food infection as well as the incidence and major symptoms. Infection control, prevention of food poisoning and sources of food contamination are identified. **Chapter 4** considers the most prevalent eating disorder in the UK (obesity). It outlines the causes, definitions and reasons why people become overweight together with clinical measurement and principles of treatment.

Module 4: Other influences on diet

Chapter 1 considers the issue of alternative nutrition and why so many people adopt this form of nutrition. It explores the concepts of health foods, organic foods, philosophical, macrobiotic and vegetarian diets. **Chapter 2** focuses on the diet of minority ethnic communities in the UK. In particular, the major religions of these ethnic groups are discussed in relation to dietary laws, beliefs, customs and eating practices. A snapshot of food selection and general health issues is included.

Module 5: Diet and the treatment of disease

This section of the textbook considers the major diseases found in clinical practice and explains in detail the nature and principles of dietary intervention or care. The practical implementation of the various dietary prescriptions is also included. Each disease is handled systematically and includes signs and symptoms, features, relevant areas of disordered or unusual pathology and rationale for treatment and management of the condition. Each disease section concludes with a commentary of practical dietary guidelines. Module 5 consists of 13 chapters.

F. Pender
N. van Kaathoven
N. van Mierlo
August 1994

Acknowledgements

The authors would like to thank the following who have kindly given their permission to reproduce their published material.

The Royal College of Midwives Trust, London.

The HEA research and development project for the National Food Selection Guide, Newport Pagnell.

The Soil Association Limited, Bristol.

Freedom Foods Ltd., Horsham.

The Telegraph plc, London.

The Sunday Telegraph Limited, London.

Ewan MacNaughton Associates, Tonbridge.

Times Newspapers Limited, London.

David Higham Associates, London.

British Heart Foundation, London.

The Scotsman, Edinburgh.

Guardian Newspapers Limited, Manchester.

The Sunday Express, London.

Health Education Board for Scotland, Edinburgh.

Ministry of Agriculture, Fisheries and Food.

Solo Syndication Limited (The Daily Mail),London.

The Flora Project for Heart Disease Prevention, London.

Caledonian Newspapers Limited, Glasgow (The Herald).

The Independent, London.

Ministry of Supply and Services, Ottawa.

Forte (UK) Limited, London

HHL Publishing, London

RUHBC, The University of Edinburgh

Contents

Module 1

FOOD, EATING BEHAVIOUR AND PRACTICES

Introduction Module 1

In this module we will discuss the significance of food and the role of the dietitian and the nurse in dietary care. The patient's perception of food plays an important role in a person's particular eating habits. For the most part, physical and psychological factors determine one's need for food and the different appetites that people have. Ideas about food are also influenced by social, cultural, and religious factors. Practically speaking, the food available or produced in an area will also govern what a person eats and how often it is eaten.

Patients' eating habits will be discussed, showing that once in hospital, many patients' eating habits and ideas about food are challenged. Firstly, the patient is restricted to the meal times as dictated by the hospital or ward. Secondly, hospital menus often provide very little variety of food, or very culture-specific food. Finally, a patient's illness may also put restrictions on what or how they eat.

The nurse and dietitian together play a very important role in helping to establish and maintain good eating habits among patients during their hospital stay. The dietitian's main priority is that patients are eating healthy, well-balanced meals. She also deals with patients' particular eating problems, whether illness-related or existing over a longer term. What approach does the dietitian take to determine whether there is an eating problem, assessing it, and attempting to correct it? The nurse is always present on the ward and therefore best able to encourage patients with eating and drinking and sometimes provide assistance. They also take note of any significant changes among an individual's eating patterns. The way in which the nurse's role interacts with that of the dietitian will also be examined.

Finally, the problem-solving approach and its six phases will be explained and discussed as an appropriate method in patient care. This method requires cooperation between the nurse and dietitian, and various aspects of this cooperation will be considered.

The significance of food and eating habits

1. Introduction

Every day we come into regular contact with food. We eat for a variety of reasons; we may desire something to eat, or we may be hungry. We may have acquired certain eating habits, we might find one thing delicious and something else revolting, we may be influenced by advertising or we may be aware that we need to take in certain nutrients.

Learning outcomes

After studying this chapter the student should be able to:
- name the three different ways in which food is important to us;
- be aware of the differences and similarities in each other's eating habits;
- state three different factors that can influence choice of food and eating habits, and give three examples for each factor;
- explain the difference between appetite and hunger.

2. The significance of food

The meaning of food differs from person to person and from one situation to another. Although food is one of the primary necessities of life, we have minds as well as bodies, and we attach entirely different meanings to the food that we eat. A meal, or even a cup of tea, may be an opportunity to take a break from daily routine. Food can mean relaxation and pleasure, though to what extent this is true varies greatly from person to person. A person who takes time to react to things will experience a meal differently from someone who is constantly under pressure and in a hurry. For a patient in a hospital, meals are often the high points of the day.

Apart from this, food can also have a social meaning. Having a meal with a group of people can mean having a good time together and be a means of communicating with each other whereas eating alone may increase a feeling of isolation (Figure 1.1.1).

Every society has its own social and cultural eating habits, and these habits determine, to a large extent, the value that is given to food and eating. Obviously, there are a number of different factors that influence when, what, and how much someone eats, and most often these factors work subconsciously.

Study activity 1

Working in small groups, discuss the following questions to discover the differences and similarities in each other's eating habits:

a. How many times a day do you eat?

Figure 1.1.1
A pleasant meal (courtesy Forte (UK) Ltd)

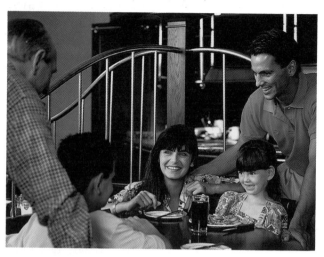

b. Is food important to you? Why or why not?
c. Do you ever eat when you are not really hungry? Why or why not?
d. Do you associate eating and drinking with having a good time?
e. Are there special eating habits or typical dishes in the area where you live?
f. What are your favourite foods?
g. Name three kinds of food you absolutely refuse to eat. Explain why.

3. Eating habits

Generally speaking, there are three groups of factors deciding choice of food and eating habits:
- physical and psychological factors
- religious, cultural and social factors
- practical circumstances.

a. Physical and psychological factors
Physical and psychological factors determine an individual's need for food, and the meaning food has for him or her. Hunger and thirst are physiological stimuli that signal the body's need for food and drink. An empty stomach or a low blood sugar level results in a feeling of hunger. We experience stomach pangs at regular intervals. It is like a biological clock that tells

us our body needs food without our consciousness having anything to do with it. Appetite, on the other hand, is a psychological stimulus that occurs at irregular intervals. Appetite may be connected with and triggered by emotional stimuli. Food is often used, for instance, as a compensation for something: as comfort, to relieve boredom, dissatisfaction or tension. It is almost as if the unpleasant feelings can be 'eaten away'.

The kinds of food you finally choose depend on their taste, appearance and aroma, on your own experience with these foods in the past, and perhaps on general ideas about their nutritional value.

Case study *Her last wish...*

Mrs Thomson was 91 years old and terminally ill. Although she was in a lot of pain she hardly ever complained, but one day she told one of the nurses that she would really love some rice pudding. She hadn't tasted it for years, but now her mouth watered when she thought of it. The nurse was sympathetic and arranged for some rice pudding to be brought as a special treat. She was then surprised when Mrs Thomson, after thoroughly enjoying her pudding, passed away peacefully.

b. *Religious, cultural and social factors*
What people eat and how they eat it is partly determined by the group, the religion or the culture they are, or want to be. Catholics, for instance, do not (or did not until recently) eat meat on Fridays or Ash Wednesday. In an Islamic society there is no place for pork, while the Hindu religion in India forbids the eating of beef. These are all food habits determined in part by religious factors.

In Britain, chips often appear on the menu, while in Italy pasta is one of the most popular foods. In Germany pork is the favourite meat dish. Many of us enjoy cockles and mussels but would not eat grasshoppers and other insects, which are commonly eaten in Africa, or snails, which are a popular delicacy in France.

Social factors sometimes can lead to eating more than you really want. For example, you may be expected to finish what is on your plate. However, in some cultures, finishing what is on your plate is the clue that you are still hungry and hence more food is brought to you. Social factors can also give food a symbolic value which may be more important than the nutritional value of the food. At a party or a meeting, for example, snacks or drinks can help people to relax and to interact socially with one another. With some people, food is used as a sign of social status or wealth and they serve expensive and exclusive foods and drinks such as pâté de foie gras, caviar, oysters, venison and champagne.

Food can also be used as an instrument of coercion as used by a hunger striker for political motives or by children who refuse to eat a meal. Children are also often rewarded or punished by means of food – usually by giving or withholding something sweet.

In modern society, many different eating patterns exist. They have changed because of growing prosperity, which has brought an overwhelming range of foodstuffs onto the market. The selection of ready-made products in supermarkets is increasing all the time and this influences the kind of food that we choose to buy. At the same time, good quality food is more appreciated and the significant growth of health food shops throughout the United Kingdom during the past decade indicates that a growing number of people are becoming more aware of, and interested in, what constitutes a healthy diet.

c. *Practical circumstances*
Practical circumstances include climate, seasonal changes, agricultural methods, food production and transport, and the degree of technology available.

In Japan, the climate is suitable for growing rice, and as a result the Japanese eat rice with most of their meals. Eskimos, on the other hand, live mainly on fish and animal meat because the extremely cold climate makes their environment unfit for agriculture. In Britain, menus differ between seasons: in summer there is a tendency to eat more cold meals and we eat fewer stews and thick soups than in winter.

In general, however, scientific advances in agricultural methods and improved re-frigerated transport have meant that the climate now plays a less significant role in the availability of what we eat and when we eat it. Thirty years ago, the availability of fruit and vegetables throughout Western Europe was governed to a large extent by the seasons whereas today there is a great and ever-increasing variety obtainable all the year round. In Third World countries there are fewer opportunities for growing, transporting or processing foodstuffs than in the Western world. There is less food available, with little or no variety, and climatic factors, such as droughts, can have devastating effects, especially in Africa, resulting in recurring famine and widespread starvation.

Study activity 2

a. Look at each group of factors influencing eating habits and decide which ones influence *your* eating behaviour.

b. Comment on the following statement:
  'For many patients, one of the most frustrating things about being ill is that their liberty to eat whenever they are hungry or feel like eating is taken away. Having breakfast at 7 a.m., lunch at 12, and tea at 5 p.m. is an ordeal for people who are used to eating more frequently and less regularly.'
c. Is it possible to change eating habits? Explain your answer.
d. Why do modern eating habits differ from those of 50 years ago?

4. Summary

We eat and drink several times a day. The meaning our food has for us, however, can differ from person to person and from situation to situation. The most basic value of food is physiological, because we eat and drink to survive, but in our society food can also be important in other ways. We often eat and drink for psychological and social reasons. Our choice of food and our eating habits are influenced by three groups of factors:

- physical and psychological factors
- religious, cultural and social factors
- practical circumstances.

These factors have been explained using a number of examples as illustrations.

The roles of the dietitian and the nurse

1. Introduction

In her working environment, a nurse will often come into contact with patients who need to be helped with eating or drinking. This help can vary from merely observing to completely taking over the responsibility of feeding the patient. Sometimes the nurse will observe a patient's eating patterns as part of her normal routine and she may assess and record intake. There is regular consultation between nurses and dietitians in a situation where a patient is prescribed a special diet or a change of diet. When a patient suffers from lack of appetite, cooperation between nurse and dietitian can be very important.

One of the most important principles for those providing food and drink is compliance with the habits and wishes of the patient whenever possible. Factors to consider are:

What would the patient like to eat and how much?

Where and how does he want to eat: in bed, at the table, alone or in company?

What foods does the patient dislike?

The extent to which these habits and wishes can be complied with will, to some extent, depend on the way meals are organised in the institution.

Learning outcomes

After studying this chapter the student should be able to:
- describe the main roles of a dietitian working in an institution;
- describe how a patient may have a diet prescribed;
- explain, using at least three examples, how a nurse can give essential support to the dietitian's work;
- describe how a nurse should oversee a patient's food and drink intake; what observations should be made and what kind of assistance can be useful.

2. The role of the dietitian working in an institution

One role of the dietitian working in an institution is to ensure that the meals provided are healthy and well-balanced. In most cases, this means giving advice when the menus are being planned. Apart from this, the dietitian advises about diets for particular patients. Where a doctor has made a diagnosis and feels that a special diet may help, the patient may be referred to a dietitian. This referral will be in writing. The dietitian or doctor or both will then decide what changes in diet will be necessary and the dietitian and the patient will formulate a diet together. The dietitian must inform the ward personnel and give instructions on how to support the patient's diet, and also advise the kitchen staff about when and how to prepare special dietary meals.

Figure 1.2.1
Phases in a problem-solving process

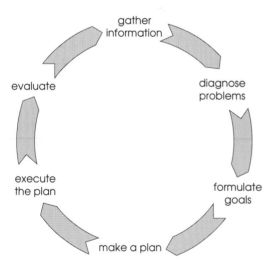

gather information

evaluate

diagnose problems

execute the plan

formulate goals

make a plan

3. Solving problems in theory and practice

One of the significant changes in health care in recent years has been the emphasis on the central role of the patient. Instead of others deciding what is best for the patient, health care workers now use a problem-solving approach to arrive at a plan for dealing with an illness or health problems through discussion and cooperation with the patient himself, focusing on the patient's wishes and symptoms.

Six different phases can be distinguished in such a problem-solving process, and these may be repeated a number of times. Figure 1.2.1 illustrates these phases and shows the cyclical nature of the problem-solving process.

Case Study *Problem-solving in theory and practice*

Mr Johnston is a 78-year-old man who was admitted to hospital with a fractured hip following a fall in the street. He is confined to bed. He is 168 cm (5 ft 6 in) tall, weighs 59 kg (9 st 4lb), is balding and has somewhat dry skin. For some days now Mr Johnston has been complaining of feeling bloated and is troubled by infrequent bowel movements. Recently, he has been eating little and has particular problems with eating hot dinners. Rather than eat sandwiches, he chooses something milky, like porridge, which he really enjoys. He does not drink a lot for fear of having to use the bedpan too often. Due to the infrequent bowel movement and the bloated feeling, a doctor is consulted. The doctor in turn consults a dietitian to see whether any assistance can be provided.

Before a dietitian can solve such a problem, the precise nature and cause of the problems have to be pinpointed. To achieve this the following actions may be taken:

Compiling information
The dietitian investigates what personal symptoms the patient may have.

Mr Johnston's symptoms are constipation, a feeling of being bloated and problems with eating hot food. The dietitian asks questions about his eating and drinking habits and takes note of his height and weight, the medication he uses and the pattern of his bowel movements. In addition, the dietitian determines the nutrients the patient requires and assesses the patient's understanding of his illness.

Determining the problem
The compiled data is analysed and evaluated. Eating habits are compared with the planned diet and the symptoms are examined in conjunction with the information which has been collected. The low intake of dietary fibre, for example, may have contributed to his symptoms.

Establishing the aims
The aims will be described in as much detail as possible so that everyone involved is aware of the intended goals and the period of time available to achieve them. For example, one goal may be that within a few weeks the frequency of bowel movements will increase.

Drawing up a plan
A plan to promote regular bowel movements is drawn up together with the patient. This might, for example, include an intake rich in dietary fibre and advice to drink more and, where possible, to take more physical exercise.

Executing a plan
The dietitian draws up a plan with the patient and informs the catering staff of the changes which are required. The dietitian will also inform the ward of the plan, requesting support where necessary. This may be recorded in nursing care plans.

Evaluation
An assessment will be made as to whether the goal has been attained. If bowel function has not improved, the dietitian and nurses must then try to pinpoint the possible reasons.

In this process, a nurse can provide important support, particularly in the compilation of information on such factors as the patient's eating habits and symptoms, and in the implementation of the plan. The nurse can, for example, assist the patient in following the appropriate diet and ensure that he drinks enough. In addition, she can discuss with the patient the best ways to vary the diet, encourage physical exercise as much as possible and try to be responsive to the patient's wishes and symptoms. Meticulous observation and reporting of the patient's appetite, drink, weight and defecation patterns are important. A nurse's observation of, for instance, whether the defecation pattern has actually improved, can also provide support in the evaluation of the plan.

4. The role of the nurse in providing dietary care

Nurses play an important role in providing dietary care on a ward. They are always in the vicinity of the patient and are best able to provide encouragement with eating and drinking. They also have the best opportunity to acquaint themselves with the patient's eating habits and needs, and to observe and report changes in appetite, body weight and drinking patterns. Where necessary, they can call upon the assistance of a dietitian to solve a dietary problem.

Often a patient requires guidance in choosing a meal or some of the separate elements of a meal, such as the type of bread, sandwich filling, or vegetables. If a patient cannot feed himself (because of serious illness or restricted movement of the hand or arm), a nurse can provide assistance (Figure 1.2.2). However, many patients do not like being helped to eat and drink. It is usually best to let the patient do as much as possible himself, and thus retain a greater feeling of independence and dignity.

Figure 1.2.2
Helping a patient to eat

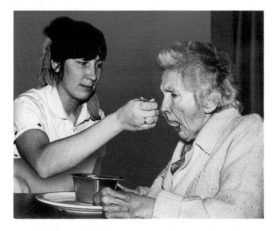

Although catering staff and dietitians are involved, the nurse also has responsibility for providing individual dietary care. We can summarise the nurse's tasks in the provision of such care as follows:

Compiling data on someone's self care with respect to eating and drinking, for example:
- How does the patient feel physically and mentally?
- What is the patient's body weight?
- Can the patient feed himself? Can he hold a cup or glass, move his arms, open sealed packets? Does he require assistance in choosing meals?
- What other aids does he require?
- Does the patient have dietary problems?
- How is the patient's appetite and desire to drink?
- How well can the patient chew?
- Can the patient bring food from home?
- Is the patient on a diet?
- How often does the patient eat, what does he eat, what are his likes and dislikes with regard to food?

During the provision of care with respect to eating and drinking, the nurse can:
- Check whether the patient is sitting or lying comfortably.
- When necessary, encourage eating, drinking, and particularly a diet which promotes health.

- Provide friendly assistance with eating and drinking and take into consideration that it can be psychologically difficult for a patient to accept help.
- Serve food and drink so that it is as attractively presented as possible and try to ensure that it does not go cold.
- Make sure that the surroundings are pleasant for dining (fresh air, quiet surroundings without doctors' calls, a nicely laid table or a clean and attractively arranged serving tray) and that the clearing up is not undertaken too quickly.
- Try to avoid monotony and routine by helping the patient to vary his choice of food and drink if necessary.
- Take eating habits, religious observances and diets into consideration.
- Provide information on healthy foods and diets in consultation with the dietitian.
- Try to maintain the patient's independence as much as possible when it comes to eating and drinking, if necessary by the use of special cutlery or other aids (Figure 1.2.3).
- Observe appetite and feelings of thirst, check the patient's body weight and note the amount of food that is left on the plate.
- Discuss adjustments to a patient's diet, for example, with a dietitian.
- If necessary maintain a fluid balance chart or record of the patient's intake.

Figure 1.2.3
Specially modified plates and cutlery

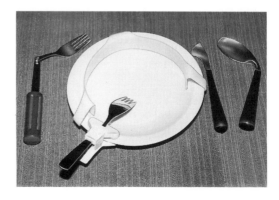

Study activity

Mrs Williams is a 59-year-old and has recently been admitted to the neurology ward in a hospital. A little over a week ago she suffered a brain haemorrhage and, as a result, is paralysed on one side. She has been put on a soft diet of porridge in the morning and a liquidised hot dinner in the afternoon. One of the diagnoses made on the ward was dehydration:
   a. What data would you have to compile to be able to make this diagnosis?
   b. Which nursing objectives could you formulate in this case?
   c. On which points of the plan is it important to involve the patient?

5. Summary

The dietitian and the nurse play the central practical roles in providing dietary care. A problem-solving approach, with its six phases, may be the most suitable method of achieving appropriate solutions for patient care. Being able to work effectively with foods and diets involves compiling data about patients' self-care with respect to eating and drinking, and carrying out a number of specific tasks during this period. Good cooperation between nursing staff and the dietitian is essential to achieve this. A nurse provides important support for the dietitian, especially in the compilation of patient data and in the execution and evaluation of a treatment programme.

Final test for Module 1

Instructions

This section consists of 12 statements. Each one may be correct or incorrect. The answer required is either YES or NO.

In your assessment of whether one of the 12 items is correct or not, you should base your decision only on the circumstances and facts given. The questions are arranged in groups, in the order that the related topics occurred in the text.

After ensuring that all the questions have been answered, check the results of the test yourself using the answers at the back of the book.

1. The only significance we attach to eating and drinking is related to the primary needs of human beings.
2. Appetite is a psychological stimulus, whereas hunger and thirst are physiological stimuli.
3. Food is sometimes used as a way of alleviating tension.
4. Nausea and headaches are social factors which can influence the choice of food.
5. Muslims do not eat lamb, for religious reasons.
6. The task of a dietitian in an institution is concerned with the provision of healthy food and special diets.
7. When a patient is referred to a dietitian for a diet, a written referral is usually required from a doctor.
8. The use of the problem-solving process allows carers who work in the health service to make individual decisions about what is most appropriate for a patient.
9. As a nurse, you can support the work of a dietitian by compiling data, by executing a nutritional care plan and assessing its success.
10. A patient or resident may have psychological problems in accepting assistance with eating and drinking.
11. Observations of a patient's appetite, thirst and body weight are not among the tasks that nurses carry out.
12. Specially modified cutlery and drinking vessels hamper the patient's independence when eating and drinking.

References and further reading

Caliendo M, (1981) *Nutrition and Preventive Health Care.* Macmillan Publishing Co., New York.

Calkins B, (1989) Florence Nightingale: on feeding an army. *American Journal of Clinical Nutrition,* 50, 1260-1265.

Hamilton E, Whitney E and Sizer F, (1991) *Nutrition: Concepts and Controversies.* 5th ed. West Publishing Co., New York.

Janes W, (1988) *Healthy Nutrition: Prevention of Nutrition-related Dseases in Europe.* WHO Publications, European Series, No.24, Copenhagen.

Keane A and Willetts A, (1994) Factors that affect food choice. *Nutrition and Food Science,* No 4, July/August, 15-17.

Leeds A , Judd P, and Lewis B, (1990) *Nutrition Matters for Practice Nurses.* J Libbey, London.

Leverkus C, Cole-Hamilton I, Gunnar K, Starr J, and Stanway A, (1985) *The Great British Diet.* Century Publishing, London.

McVicker R, (1994) Healthful eating: the food industry role. *Nutrition Today,* 29, No 1, 37-38.

Mahan K and Arlin A, (1992) *Krause's Food, Nutrition and Diet Therapy.* 8th ed. W B Saunders Co., Philadelphia.

National Consumer Council, (1992) *Your Food: Whose Choice?* HMSO, London,

Wardlaw G and Insel P. (1990) *Perspectives in Nutrition.* 2nd ed. Mosby, St Louis.

Wells D, (1990) What do doctors know about nutrition? *Nutrition and Food Science,* No 4, March/April 14-16.

Whitney E and Rolfes S, (1993) *Understanding Nutrition.* 6th ed. West Publishing Co., New York.

Module 2

NUTRITION AND HEALTH

Introduction Module 2

In Module One, we examined the significance of food and the roles of the dietitian and nurse in dietary care. The physical and psychological aspects of nutrition were considered and discussed. In this module we are primarily concerned with the question of why nutrition is important for our physical health. In reality, of course, physical, mental and social welfare cannot be considered separately because they continually influence each other.

It is estimated that during our lifetime we each consume some 35 tons (35,000 kg) of food, and this enormous mountain of food must be processed in the body. What effects do the various components of this food have on a person's health? When can a diet really be considered healthy?

Never before has the choice of foodstuffs been so great and so varied. How do we, as consumers, know what is good for us? The basic principles of dietetics are discussed and although there are various theories, the view discussed here is the one which is presently the most widely accepted. We will examine some of the factors which need to be considered when constructing or evaluating a diet using tools such as the food guide. The labels on packaged foods can provide some useful information. Some attention will also be paid to the protective measures set by the Government to ensure the safety of foodstuffs.

A separate chapter deals with nutrition in various stages of life. Food intake has a continuing influence on a person's health throughout life, and health in later life is partially determined by the food which has been consumed early on in life. For instance, osteoporosis among the elderly may partly be attributed to a very low consumption of dairy products in earlier years. A variety of circumstances can persuade us to eat the kinds of food which may not meet the requirements of a healthy diet and some of these influences on what we choose to eat will be considered.

The influence of nutrition on the body

1. Introduction

Although nutrition can have a great deal of influence on the mental and social welfare of a person, in this chapter we are going to focus on the significance of nutrition on the body. Nutrition determines the normal operation of many of the mechanisms in our body and the correct quantity of nutrients and energy in the diet is essential for the maintenance of health. Deficiencies or surpluses will have a detrimental influence on the proper functioning of the body.

Learning outcomes

After studying this chapter the student should be able to:
- explain what a healthy diet is in terms of nutrients;
- describe what nutrients are;
- describe the functions of fuelling, building and regulating substances;
- name two fuelling substances, two regulating substances and three building substances;
- describe the concept of good nutritional status;
- describe the characteristics of malnutrition, overeating and an unbalanced diet and give an example of each of these concepts.

2. What nutrition means for the body

When can one actually speak of a healthy diet for the body? Although there are various views, in this chapter we will restrict ourselves to the definition which the profession of dietetics mainly uses, namely that a healthy diet is one which includes the appropriate quantities of all the substances the body needs (other views will be discussed in Module 4, Chapter 1).

At present, we know of over 50 substances which our bodies require in order to function efficiently. These are known as nutrients; proteins, fats, carbohydrates, vitamins, minerals and water are the most important ones. They are present in foodstuffs such as bread, cheese and fruit (Figure 2.1.1). One food product usually contains several nutrients. For example, fruit contains vitamin C and carbohydrates. However, there is no one food product which contains all the nutrients. That is why one food product alone can never be called 'healthy'. One cannot say that an orange is healthy, because eating ten oranges a day and nothing else would result in an unbalanced diet. The quality of a healthy diet, therefore, is determined by the total range of foodstuffs consumed over days or weeks.

Figure 2.1.1
Important foodstuffs

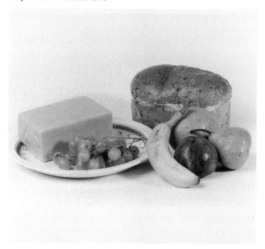

Some foods contain few or no nutrients, such as coffee, tea, alcohol, cocoa, spices, herbs and salt. We consume them for pleasure, only because they smell or taste good (Figure 2.1.2).

Nutrients have various functions in our body as follows:

– **providing energy**. Our body is constantly using energy for internal and external effort and to maintain body temperature. Energy is used internally for breathing, thinking and maintaining heart and kidney function. External effort includes such activities as walking, cycling, standing and writing. Carbohydrates and fats are important sources of energy. They are called fuelling substances and their energy content is expressed in kilojoules or kilocalories.

– **building up and restoring tissue such as muscles, the nervous system and bones.** Proteins, minerals and water, the building substances, are the key nutrients in this process.

– **helping with the proper functioning of processes in the body such as fighting off illness and infection.** Vitamins and minerals, the regulating substances, play the main role here.

Chapter 3 will deal in more detail with the role of the most important nutrients in our daily diet.

Figure 2.1.2
Items with little or
no nutritional value

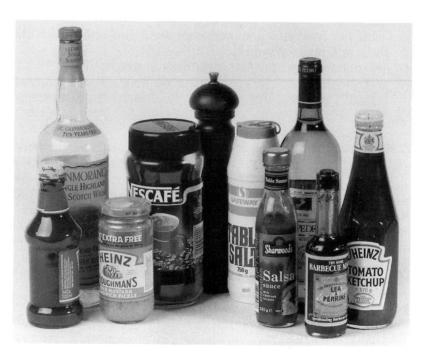

3. The quantity and quality of nutrition

The ultimate goal of eating and drinking is maintaining or achieving sound nutritional status. A working definition of good nutritional status is when a person's diet contains sufficient nutrients and energy, and that these substances are properly absorbed and metabolised by the body.

One indication of good nutritional status is a body weight which is in correct proportion to height. Another indicator is elastic skin, which has been pinched between your fingers and then becomes smooth again immediately upon being released. However, using body weight and skin elasticity as the only criteria can be misleading. It is only possible to form a true picture of dietary status by observing the eating behaviour of a patient and by checking against all the signs listed in Figure 2.1.4. Laboratory analysis can also offer valuable aid in such evaluations.

Figure 2.1.3
© The Scotsman 28/6/93

Sweet talk that aims to bear fruit

by Bryan Christie
Health Correspondent

SCOTS are being encouraged to give up sugary snacks and get their teeth into healthier alternatives in a drive to improve eating habits.

Advertising posters will go up across the country from today in an attempt to persuade people to eat more fruit. The message is delivered with humour but the intent is deadly serious.

Emerging evidence suggests that people who have a high intake of fruit and vegetables are at much lower risk of contracting heart disease and cancer than those whose consumption is low.

The problem in Scotland is that too few people eat enough fruit. A survey conducted among 1,000 people in the west of Scotland found that almost a quarter of people had fruit less than once a week and never in the winter. Only one person in 20 ate fruit and green vegetables daily.

By comparison, the World Health Organisation recommends everyone to eat five portions of fruit and vegetables a day. A portion equals an apple, banana or a serving of carrots or peas.

The Health Education Board for Scotland has investigated people's attitudes to fruit and vegetables to find out how consumption can be increased. Martin Raymond, the Board's Deputy Director of Programmes, said: "There is a sort of folk understanding – an apple a day keeps the doctor away – that kind of thing. The trouble is fruit is seen as being a bit dull. We are trying to show it in a new light."

The campaign features the everyday and the exotic. Mr Raymond said market-testing of the advertisements showed that those featuring the exotic fruits were very well received.

The advertising posters will be going up in about 700 bus shelters. They are also being reproduced in a smaller form for use in general practitioner surgeries and in community centres.

Vegetables are every bit as important as fruit but the Board found there was a reluctance among the public to use them for snacks. That view was best summed up by one Lanarkshire respondent. "I think the good people of Coatbridge would think I'd gone round the twist if I was sitting at my desk and I pulled out a carrot to chew on."

Figure 2.1.4
Signs of poor nutritional status

1. Weight loss (5% in one month or more than 10% in 6 months*)
2. Muscle atrophy
3. Loss of subcutaneous fat tissue
4. Fluid retention**
5. Apathy, fatigue and irritability
6. Signs of vitamin and mineral deficiencies in skin, hair, eyes, mouth, tongue, bones, nervous system, mucous membranes of mouth and eyes (see Module 2, Chapter 3)
7. Susceptibility to infections

* The patient may still be overweight in some cases.
** For example, in patients with infections, traumas or burns. These can cause a large amount of body protein to be broken down in a very short period of time. This leads to a low serum albumin concentration, which, in turn, results in oedema.

In hospital, patients are at risk of having an unsatisfactory nutritional status. This can have important medical consequences, including weight loss, poor healing of wounds, greater risk of infections, fatigue, greater risk of diarrhoea and increased risk during operations. Poor nutritional status occurs particularly among patients with fever, infections, cancer, after major operations, in burns cases, with the use of certain medicines (such as corticosteroids and antibiotics), where there are problems with swallowing or chewing, where there are wounds and tumours in the gastrointestinal tract and among patients suffering from depression or anxiety.

Figure 2.1.5
Malnutrition

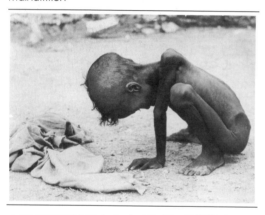

Malnutrition, overeating, and an unbalanced diet can all jeopardise a person's nutritional status.

a. Malnutrition
It has been calculated that more than half of the world's population suffers from mild to moderate malnutrition. Malnutrition is caused by insufficient food intake (Figure 2.1.5). Every day hundreds of people die of starvation, particularly in the developing countries. This is a result of, among other things, poverty, inadequate distribution of food, poor farming land, poor seed, unfavourable climatic factors and transport problems.

Malnutrition occurs in the West as the result of poverty, stress or excessive alcohol consumption. According to one estimate, 2.5% of the population in the industrialised countries eat less than their minimum requirements (Figure 2.1.6).

We can distinguish three types of malnutrition: insufficient energy, insufficient protein and insufficient vitamins and/or minerals. Often there is a combination of nutritional deficiencies. This classification of malnutrition suggests that malnourished people are not always too thin. Overweight people can also suffer from malnutrition if they have an unbalanced diet. This can result in a dietary deficiency of essential nutrients, causing greater susceptibility to infection, a slower recovery from illness and so on.

Figure 2.1.6
© The Independent 6/11/92

Poor People suffer unhealthy diet and days without food

Oliver Gillie

Young people in Britain who are out of work frequently starve for up to three days at a time.

Pregnant teenagers have a high rate of miscarriage caused by having insufficient to eat, and mothers living on benefit often go without food so their children will not starve, according to a report by the National Consumer Council.

It is impossible for children and teenagers to obtain sufficient food with current Department of Social Security allowances, the report says. The allowance provides them not only with a poorly balanced diet but with insufficient food for energy and insufficient protein for growth.

Contrary to popular belief, poor people buy more sensibly – getting more nutrients per penny – than those who are better off. To get the nutrients they need at a price they can afford their diet tends to be high in fats and sugar. A packet of crisps, for example, will give 100 calories of energy for 12p and two custard cream biscuits will give as much energy for 3p.

A healthier choice such as a medium banana would cost 20p and three small apples 29p.

The high level of saturated fats and lack of fresh green vegetables in the diets of poor people make them vulnerable to cancer and heart disease in later life, the National Consumer Council says.

A healthy diet costs £11.71 per person per week on average and could cost as little as £10 a week, according to the Ministry of Agriculture, Fisheries and Food. To conform to such a diet, however, poor families would have to cut out meat almost entirely, double their consumption of breakfast cereals and eat five times as much wholemeal bread, the National Consumer Council says. It would mean eating eight slices of bread a day – five of which would be dry, the other three with a thin scraping of margarine.

The trend towards large superstores away from high streets has increased the problems of poor people who generally cannot afford the fares to reach them. The cost of food in corner shops, however, is at least 20 per cent more than in supermarkets.

Poor women with children cut down on their own food, living on tea and toast for days at a time, in order to give their children enough. According to one study quoted by the National Consumer Council, a quarter of women on low incomes fall below deficiency levels for eight essential nutrients.

The Family Welfare Association has found that 47 per cent of families asking for help did not have enough money for food after paying for rent, fuel and other necessities. More than half were £10 a week short. In another survey, by the National Children's Home, parents in one out of five families and children in one out of ten families had gone hungry in the last month.

But most vulnerable of all are homeless young people under 25 who are entitled to minimum benefits or none at all. Their daily intake of energy is one third of what it should be, with major deficiencies in vitamins, iron, protein and calcium. Most 16- and 17-year-olds have no guaranteed support. They have frequent long spells without food; one to three days is normal, the National Consumer Council says. *Your Food: Whose Choice?* HMSO; London, £10.95.

b. Overeating

In the West overeating is a far more common problem (Figure 2.1.7). This is particularly the case in countries with an affluent population and an overabundant supply of food. Obesity occurs when the energy intake is too high and energy expenditure is too low. A diet with an excess of proteins, vitamins and minerals also has an unfavourable effect on the body (see also Chapter 3 of this module).

Figure 2.1.7
Exercise can help to lose weight

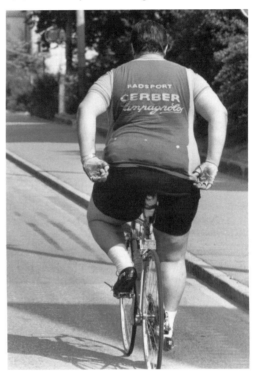

c. Unbalanced diet

When we speak of an unbalanced diet, we are referring to a diet which usually contains a sufficient amount of energy, but which is lacking in quality, in other words, a diet which does not contain all the nutrients a person needs. One example might be a child who eats nothing but sweets or junk food, and thus does not get enough vitamins and minerals. Elderly people sometimes eat insufficient fruit and vegetables, resulting in a vitamin C deficiency. Overzealous dieting also compromises nutritional status.

Study activity

1. Try to think of other examples of an unbalanced diet.
2. Why do you think many millions of pounds are spent every year on convenience foods?
3. Write down what you eat and drink over the course of one day, from the moment you get up to the moment you go to bed. Try to write down everything as precisely as possible. For example, note the type of bread and butter, margarine or low fat spread you eat, and the sort of cheese or cold meat you select. When you are having a hot meal, count how many spoonfuls of vegetables, potatoes and gravy you are taking and note the kind of meat or fish, whether butter, margarine or oil has been used in preparing the meal and how the vegetables have been prepared and don't forget any starter or pudding. Try to give a precise account of any snacks taken in between meals as well. Pinpoint any weaknesses in your diet that might lead to poor nutrient intake.

4. Summary

The physiological effects of nutrition only take place after food has been absorbed and metabolised. A human being needs over 50 nutrients in order to function properly. Patients in hospitals or nursing homes can have poor nutritional status. This can have important medical consequences. You can form a picture of a patient's nutritional status by observing his eating behaviour and checking whether he shows any of the signs mentioned in Figure 2.1.4.

A healthy diet

1. Introduction

Various informational models are used to answer the question of what constitutes a healthy diet and these form useful tools for compiling and evaluating a diet. In some countries, national nutrition agencies or government offices also offer advice on how to put together a balanced diet.

Making the right choice is not always easy with new products continually coming onto the market. This means that there is an increasingly large supply of foodstuffs which can be preserved longer, are more convenient to use, or just look better. However, industrial processing can adversely influence nutritional value by adding items such as sugar, fats, and salt. The number of additives in foodstuffs is also increasing, with various advantages and disadvantages. The labels on packaging offer valuable information in this respect. In this chapter we will look at the meanings of various words and symbols which appear on food packaging and discuss some of the legislation and regulations which apply to the provision of food.

Learning outcomes

After studying this chapter the student should be able to:
- describe the changes in eating habits since the 1950s;
- state which foodstuffs might appear in a typical food guide and in which sections they appear;
- give ten recommendations for a healthy diet;
- describe the most important rules for using the food guide;
- describe why nutritional variation is necessary;
- compile a one-day menu and put together a meal according to the principles of the food guide;
- explain why some products in the food guide are to be preferred to others from the same group;
- explain why the food guide has been presented in four groups, and give several examples;
- explain the portion guide that determines the number and size of servings for different population groups;
- list some advantages and disadvantages of using additives in foodstuffs;

– explain the value of the Food and Safety Act;
– know which information, by law, must appear on the labels of packaged foodstuffs.

Study activity 1

Discuss the following questions in small groups. Compare each other's opinions and then inform the entire group of the results.

a. Nutrition and diet are often the topics of discussion on radio and television, and in newspapers and magazines. Usually the discussion involves the unhealthy eating habits of the Western world. Do you think there is something wrong with our current eating habits? Explain why.

b. Can lack of nutrition play a part in the occurrence of illness?

c. Have you ever changed your eating habits?

Figure 2.2.1
Nature's diet for health

Wild foods hold clues to health

THE DIET of wild plants, flowers and fruits enjoyed by our ape-like ancestors holds clues to the cause of diet-related health problems, a professor told the meeting.

Today's Western foods may not be as nutritious as those of non-human primates, said Prof Katharine Milton.

"Plant domestication, food additives and food processing may make many of the foods we eat today quite different from those our bodies evolved to handle," she said.

Today fast foods and overwhelming variety in diet, particularly in the Western nations, have left people confused about what to eat.

Looking at the nutritional content of wild plant foods may suggest factors underlying many current health problems, said Prof Milton.

"The chemical composition of these wild plant foods may have much to tell us about the ways in which our modern diets have become out of step with our biology."

For example, working with colleagues she found that the leaves and fruits eaten by wild monkeys are high in vitamin C and that monkeys consume hundreds of milligrams each day.

Moreover these wild plant foods contain a great deal of pectin, which attacks cholesterol – possibly reducing the risk of blocked arteries – and dietary fibre, thought to combat colon cancer.

"The tropical forests are a natural dietary laboratory which we have thus far failed to utilise," said Prof Milton.

2. Changes in eating habits

Since the 1950s our eating habits have undergone quite substantial changes. More foodstuffs are continually appearing on the market with more than 8,000 different products now available. In addition, people can generally spend more money on food and drink than they could before the 1950s. As a result, we are eating more of some foodstuffs and less of others. For example, we are eating almost twice as much meat and cheese, but less bread and fewer potatoes. In particular, the consumption of sugar has increased dramatically. A hundred years ago we consumed about 2 kg of sugar per person annually, whilst now we may consume as much as 35 kg a year (the average is 9 kg). Our intake of sugar comes from that added to coffee, tea, sweets and cakes, as well as from the processed sugar which is present in all sorts of sauces and products in tins, cartons and jars.

These changes in eating habits have had significant consequences for our health and the increase in the amount and variety of food available has been accompanied by an increase in many diseases which seldom occurred in the past. A healthy diet can help to prevent the diseases connected with the excesses of the Western diet (see Module 3, Chapter 1).

Figure 2.2.2
© The Scotsman, 10/7/91

Boycott the biscuit tin feast on fruit, says report

Chocolate bars and fizzy drinks are all right in moderation, it is claimed but it seems we are not moderate enough

SWEET-TOOTHED Britain was urged yesterday to curb its passion for sugary foods as the Government gave its own diet plan advice for the Nineties. The craving for fatty dishes should be reduced, said the report on healthy eating.

The report said Britons should cut down on fizzy drinks, cakes and biscuits, and eat more cherries, grapes, potatoes and bread.

According to the report, eating a Mars bar, which contains the equivalent of five teaspoons of sugar, and drinking a can of Coke, which has eight teaspoons, would put a person over the average daily recommended amount of 12 teaspoons. A teaspoon contains 5 grams of sugar.

The health message is a familiar one but it is backed by what Health Secretary William Waldegrave hailed as the world's most comprehensive and up-to-date study on nutrition and diet.

He said at the publication of the 200-page study the Government's aim was not to provide the recipe for the perfect diet, but professional nutritionists and everyone else now had all the details needed for good advice on healthy eating.

Consumer and health groups welcomed the report but said Government action was needed to put the recommendations into effect.

The study, from the Committee on the Medical Aspects of Food gives advice on 33 nutrients and forms of food energy, including a range of vitamins.

In particular, Britain should be eating less refined sugar, the type spooned into coffee and tea as well as used in a wide range of manufactured food.

The report endorses warnings that sugar is a major cause of tooth decay, although the Sugar Bureau, the voice of the industry, insisted the document had acknowledged the evidence was "scanty". At present, the average person is getting 13 to 14 per cent of his or her total energy from refined sugar, about 15 teaspoons a day.

That should be cut to about 10 per cent of total energy intake – about 12 spoonfuls.

Most of the sugar eaten comes in fizzy drinks, cakes confectionery and biscuits so the message is to cut down, but not eliminate, those foods in the diet.

Fatty foods, including most take-away meals, meat without the fat trimmed off, butter, cheese, cream, many snacks, cakes and biscuits should be cut from 40 per cent of energy intake to 35 per cent.

In particular, saturated fat – the type found in animal products like meat and dairy foods – should be cut to the current average of 16 per cent of total energy intake to 11 per cent.

We should also eat less salt, more calcium – found in milk, cheese and bread – and more vitamin C, with fruit, vegetables, including potatoes, being good sources, said the report.

Fibre, found in fruit, cereals and vegetables, should form a substantially bigger part of the average diet with consumption stepped up from 11 grams a day to 18.

The panel that produced the report was chaired by the Government's chief medical officer, Sir Donald Acheson. He said: "The importance of this report lies in its comprehensive coverage – not just the energy required for life but also of the desirable contributions to that energy from the various fats, carbo-hydrates and proteins, as well as vitamins and minerals."

He said the target figures set in the report would be expected to reduce the burden of illness and death from a number of diseases related to diet, including coronary heart disease and some cancers.

The report contains numerous tables setting out estimated average requirements for energy. A man aged 19 to 50 is said to require 2,550 calories a day, while a woman at the same age needs only 1,940. A man aged 75 and over needs 2,100 calories and a woman of that age 1,810.

The Sugar Bureau said the report would end a campaign of deliberate misinformation waged against the trade over recent weeks. It insisted the report made clear that for most of the population there is absolutely no need to reduce sugar consumption.

"The committee recommends only a tiny reduction in sugar consumption against current average population intake for the sake of dental health, although the committee accepts there is only 'scanty evidence' for this," it claimed.

Michael Shersby, Conservative MP for Uxbridge, who is parliamentary adviser to the bureau, said: "The sugar industry does not accept that total energy intake from sugar should be reduced at all, because there is no credible scientific evidence to back such a recommendation."

The Consumers' Association said the study should end any confusion about what constituted a healthy diet, but its scientific jargon must be translated into easy-to-understand advice.

The shadow health secretary, Robin Cook, asked if the Government was tough enough to meet the standards set by the study. "Will health ministers demand clear labelling so that consumers can tell which foods are high in sugar and fat? Will they ask their colleagues at the Ministry of Agriculture to stop subsidising the wrong foods?"

The Coronary Prevention Group welcomed the report but said the Government must act by introducing practical policies.

Steps needed included urgent guidelines for school meals and other catering outlets as three in four children ate too much saturated fat.

Study activity 2

Using the above information, can you establish which nutrients in our diets are likely to be in excess of our needs and which ones we are likely to be lacking?

3. Food guides

There are various organisations within the United Kingdom which provide healthy eating advice, some of them with government support. In addition, dietetic departments at local hospitals or community dietitians also give advice on good dietary habits. Most information is based upon principles described in food guides. Recent publications (*Health of the Nation 1992* and *The Scottish Diet 1993*) have made recommendations or suggested dietary goals based upon findings that our national diet is poor and could be improved by adoption of country-wide dietary guidelines. The information which is given should allow for a diet which is affordable and which takes account of our industrialised society.

The general principles of healthy eating are widely recognised and the following ten recommendations (applicable to everyone over one year old) give guidance for selection of a healthy balanced diet.

1. Eat a varied diet.
2. Eat fat in moderation.
3. Eat plenty of starch and dietary fibre.
4. Eat three meals a day, and do not have more than four snacks between them.
5. Use salt sparingly.
6. Drink at least 1.5 litres of fluid a day, and drink alcohol only in moderation.
7. Keep your weight within an acceptable range.
8. Prevent food poisoning by ensuring proper food handling and appropriate hygiene.
9. Remember the possible presence of harmful substances.
10. Read the information printed on food packaging.

The first and last recommendation will be explained in more detail in this chapter. The underlying principles of recommendations 2 to 7, and how these can be implemented, are discussed in Chapter 3 of this module. Recommendations 8 and 9 are dealt with in Module 3, Chapter 3.

By eating a varied diet, it is possible to obtain all the nutrients essential for good health. There is no single food product that contains all the necessary substances in sufficient quantity. There is only one exception – and that is breast milk – which provides all the necessary nutrients but only for the first few months of life. A food selection guide can therefore be useful in making the correct choices for daily food intake. Figure 2.2.3 shows such a guide from Canada. In this chart foodstuffs have been divided into four groups, and by selecting products from these groups daily it is possible to compile a healthy diet.

Many countries use a food selection guide to provide a consistent nutrition education message to the general public. A number of informational models exist to summarise the main food groups, the foods that are in them, and the proportion that form a balanced diet. America uses a pyramid, Canada the rainbow (described below) and the UK is to use a plate model.

In the UK, the 'Nutrition Task Force' considered that a "pictorial food selection guide would be helpful in providing consumers with simple, practical and realistic guidance for selecting a balanced diet". The project to devise such a guide involved wide consultation with representatives of professional groups, government, industries involved in preparing and selling food and those involved in nutrition education. Collaboration has resulted in the production of the national food selection guide launched in July, 1994.

The guide (Figure 2.2.4) depicts a balanced diet using a plate. The model consists of five food groups (Bread, other cereals and potatoes; Fruit and vegetables; Meat, fish and alternatives; Milk and dairy foods; Fatty and sugary foods).

The principles for the use of this guide are similar to the Canadian Food Guide described earlier.

The foodstuffs in each group in the Canadian guide are consistent with each other in the type of nutrients they contain. Those in Group 1 are particularly rich in starch and dietary fibre; Group 2 contains the products which are primarily rich in the vitamins; Group 3 contains a great deal of calcium and protein and the products in Group 4 are rich in protein and fat. A varied choice within each section is important because no single item within one section can completely replace the others. Thus, although milk as a source of protein can be replaced with meat or fish, these are no substitute as regards a source of calcium. Whilst Brussels sprouts provide a lot of vitamin C but little iron, spinach contains a lot of iron but very little vitamin C. Carrots and green cabbage are rich in carotene whilst cauliflower and cabbage provide none at all. Vegetables and fruit can also, therefore, only provide partial substitutes for each other.

In this food guide, specific attention is drawn to the relative proportions of the various foods to be consumed. The guide depicts a rainbow of foods. The outer edge which illustrates grain products occupies the most space and therefore indicates that consumption of starchy foods should be relatively high. The innermost arc illustrating meat products occupies the smallest area and thus indicates that the

intake of protein-containing foods should be comparatively lower.

For general health and the prevention of illnesses related to the excesses of the Western diet, certain foodstuffs are to be preferred to other products within the same group of the food guide. Some contain more fats and sugar or fewer vitamins and minerals than others. Additional guidance on appropriate selections within each of the four categories is also given in Figure 2.2.5.

Study activity 3

Draw up your typical day's menu or choose a hospital day's menu. Divide the foodstuffs into three groups: products which should make up the greatest part of a balanced diet, products which should be consumed in moderation and those which should be consumed relatively rarely. Using the food guide, make a judgement on the rough balance of the menu.

Requirements for different nutrients vary greatly for people of different ages, sex, and occupations. Therefore, in addition to providing information on types of food to select, the food guide also suggests the amounts of food to be eaten from the food groups (Figure 2.2.5). In general, the number of servings will increase as nutrient requirements increase. Thus, different people need different amounts of food. Examples of this appear in Figure 2.2.6.

The food guide has been written to incorporate a wide variety of tastes and food preferences so within each food group there is scope for individuals to improve their diet. For example, white and brown bread appear in group 1, the grain product group. The preferred healthy choice would be the brown bread. Further examples on guidance for food selection from the guide are included (Figure 2.2.7).

Figure 2.2.3
Canada's Food Guide

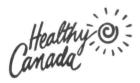

 Health and Welfare Canada   Santé et Bien-être social Canada

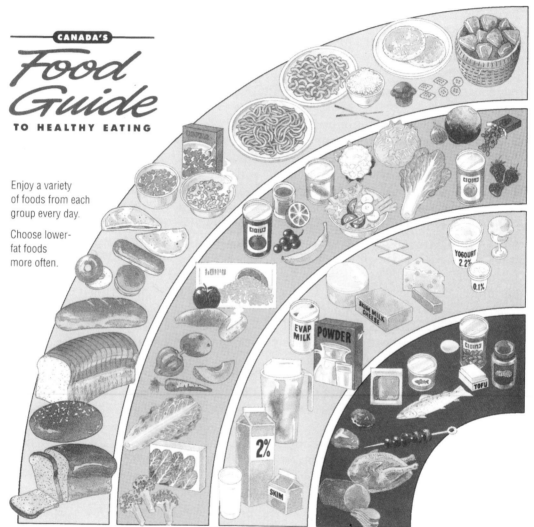

Enjoy a variety of foods from each group every day.

Choose lower-fat foods more often.

Grain Products
Choose whole grain and enriched products more often.

Vegetables & Fruit
Choose dark green and orange vegetables and orange fruit more often.

Milk Products
Choose lower-fat milk products more often.

Meat & Alternatives
Choose leaner meats, poultry and fish, as well as dried peas, beans and lentils more often.

Figure 2.2.4
The Balance of Good Health: the UK food selection guide

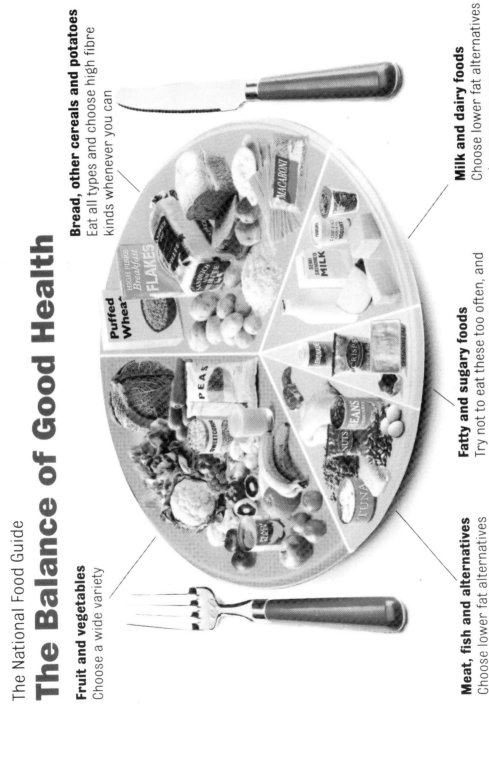

The National Food Guide

The Balance of Good Health

Bread, other cereals and potatoes
Eat all types and choose high fibre
kinds whenever you can

Milk and dairy foods
Choose lower fat alternatives
whenever you can

Fatty and sugary foods
Try not to eat these too often, and
when you do, have small amounts

Fruit and vegetables
Choose a wide variety

Meat, fish and alternatives
Choose lower fat alternatives
whenever you can

Figure 2.2.5
The Canadian Food Guide: different people need different amounts of food

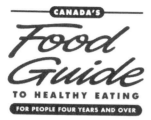

CANADA'S
Food Guide
TO HEALTHY EATING
FOR PEOPLE FOUR YEARS AND OVER

Different People Need Different Amounts of Food

The amount of food you need every day from the 4 food groups and other foods depends on your age, body size, activity level, whether you are male or female and if you are pregnant or breast-feeding. That's why the Food Guide gives a lower and higher number of servings for each food group. For example, young children can choose the lower number of servings, while male teenagers can go to the higher number. Most other people can choose servings somewhere in between.

Grain Products
5-12
SERVINGS PER DAY

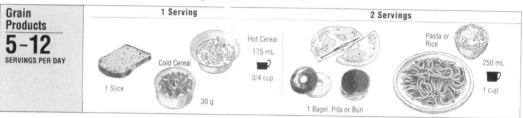

1 Serving — 1 Slice — Cold Cereal 30 g — Hot Cereal 175 mL 3/4 cup

2 Servings — 1 Bagel, Pita or Bun — Pasta or Rice 250 mL 1 cup

Vegetables & Fruit
5-10
SERVINGS PER DAY

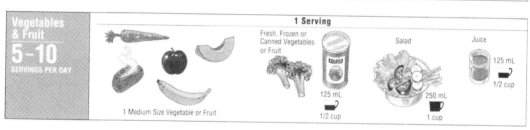

1 Serving — 1 Medium Size Vegetable or Fruit — Fresh, Frozen or Canned Vegetables or Fruit 125 mL 1/2 cup — Salad 250 mL 1 cup — Juice 125 mL 1/2 cup

Milk Products
SERVINGS PER DAY
Children 4–9 years: 2–3
Youth 10–16 years: 3–4
Adults: 2–4
Pregnant & Breast-feeding
Women: 3–4

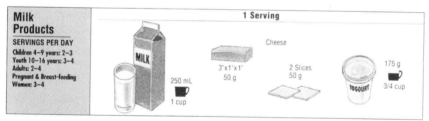

1 Serving — MILK 250 mL 1 cup — Cheese 3"x1"x1" 50 g — 2 Slices 50 g — 175 g 3/4 cup

Other Foods

Taste and enjoyment can also come from other foods and beverages that are not part of the 4 food groups. Some of these foods are higher in fat or Calories, so use these foods in moderation.

Meat & Alternatives
2-3
SERVINGS PER DAY

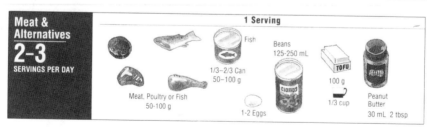

1 Serving — Meat, Poultry or Fish 50-100 g — Fish 1/3–2/3 Can 50–100 g — 1-2 Eggs — Beans 125-250 mL — TOFU 100 g — Peanut Butter 1/3 cup 30 mL 2 tbsp

Figure 2.2.6
Marie, David, Louise

How many servings from each food group do I need?

Because different people need different amounts of food, the bar side of the Food Guide suggests the following number of servings:

Grain Products **5-12** SERVINGS PER DAY	**Vegetables & Fruit** **5-10** SERVINGS PER DAY
Milk Products **2-4** SERVINGS PER DAY Children 4–9 years: 2–3 servings/day Youth 10–16 years: 3–4 servings/day Adults: 2–4 servings/day Pregnant & Breast-feeding Women: 3–4 servings/day	**Meat & Alternatives** **2-3** SERVINGS PER DAY

The number of servings you need every day from the 4 food groups and other foods depends on your age, body size, activity level, whether you are male or female and if you are pregnant or breast-feeding.

Most people will need to have more than the lower number of servings, especially pregnant and breast-feeding women, male teenagers and highly active people.

Different People Need Different Amounts of Food

Here are some examples of how people could choose their servings in one day.

FOOD PRODUCTS	MARIE	SERVINGS	DAVID	SERVINGS	LOUISE	SERVINGS
Grain Products	Marie is **5 years** old. To meet her nutrient and energy needs, Marie has the smallest number of servings from each food group and adds 'other foods'. As she grows or is more active, Marie may choose more servings.	5	David is **17** and a competitive swimmer. To meet his nutrient and energy needs, David chooses the largest number of servings from each of the 4 food groups and adds 'other foods'. David has higher energy needs than most people and at times he may need to choose **even more** servings than those shown here.	12	Louise is **35** and not very active. Like most people, she eats different amounts of food from day to day to satisfy her nutrient and energy needs. As her appetite and activity level change, Louise may adjust the number of servings and amount of 'other foods' she eats.	6
Vegetables & Fruit		5		10		7
Milk Products		2		4		2
Meat & Alternatives		2		3		2
'Other Foods'						

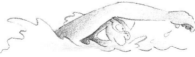
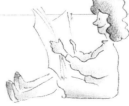

Figure 2.2.7
Examples of food selection guidance

Preferred choice

Group No.		
1	brown bread, brown crispbread, brown rice
2	fresh vegetables, fresh fruit
3	low fat dairy products
4	lean meat, pulses, fish and poultry

In moderation

Group No.		
1	white bread, biscuits, white rice
2	tinned vegetables, tinned fruit, frozen vegetables
3	medium fat dairy products
4	medium fat meat

To be avoided/eaten very infrequently

Group No.		
1	pies, cakes, croissants
2	dried vegetables
3	full fat dairy products
4	fatty meat

4. Changes in food spending

In recent years, there has been a tendency towards healthier eating habits. One useful guide to the average British diet is the annual survey carried out by the Ministry of Agriculture, Fisheries and Food. Representatives of the department question over 7,000 households to evaluate changing trends in food consumption.

By 1991, the report of the National Food Survey Committee, *Household Food Consumption and Expenditure* (HMSO), was beginning to give encouraging details of healthier eating. It showed, for example, that spending on food generally rose by 4.7 per cent (to £12.69 per person per week) and within that total the proportion spent on fruit and vegetables had also risen.

The consumption of meat rose during the year, with sales of lamb and beef increasing more than enough to compensate for a reduction in demand for pork. Skimmed and semi-skimmed milk was also rising in popularity. Almost half the households participating in the survey bought one or the other in the week during which the survey took place, and consumption of whole cream milk continued to drop in line with previous trends.

One of the most marked changes in buying patterns was the enormous rise in the sales of low fat and dairy spreads, reducing the use of butter. Sales of these spreads had risen by 50 per cent over the previous four years.

Potato consumption rose despite the fact that fewer fresh potatoes were being bought by consumers. Instead, processed potato products, from snack products to frozen chips, accounted for the increase. The amount of fresh green vegetables bought in the shops decreased by almost 7 per cent. Paradoxically, however, spending on green vegetables increased by 10 per cent. The discrepancy is explained by the trend amongst consumers to more exotic and expensive green produce such as broccoli and leaf salads.

Egg consumption also showed an increase, although it was very small, with each person in the survey eating an average of 2.25 eggs per week. The rise in cholesterol level thus indicated, however, was more than compensated by the welcome shift towards healthier eating shown by other factors in the survey.

Study activity 4

a. Put together a day's menu for yourself, choosing one or more foods or food products from each group in the food guide. Bear in mind the quantity of foodstuffs which are recommended for the daily diet of someone your age.

b. Compare this day's menu with the three groups of food you made in the Study Activity 3. Have you chosen the right kinds of food?

c. Describe in your own words why a varied diet is so important. A varied diet is easy to follow with the help of the food guide. How do you use it?

d. There are people who think the use of low fat margarine is pointless. Can you think of their reasons for this? What is your opinion?

5. Additives in our food

When we speak of the quality of our food we are not only referring to the nutritional value, but also the appearance, colour, smell, and taste of the food. For various reasons, these days, additives are used when food is prepared in factories. These additives make the food more tasty, more colourful, more aromatic, spicier, or easier to handle. All in all, the final product appears to be of a better quality, and this is reflected in sales. Over time, the consumer has become accustomed to the red colour of strawberry jam, the delicate orange of peach yoghurt and the smooth skin of unblemished fruit. You might ask yourself whether this is really necessary. For example, consider the anti-caking substances added to salt or icing sugar to make it free running; in the old days people just put a few grains of rice in the salt shaker. Aroma, colour and flavour enhancers are often used to suggest that a lot of fruit has been incorporated in desserts and sauces. The use of additives often conceals the moderate quality of the raw materials used and this negative aspect of additives needs to be recognised.

Additives can also have a positive effect. Preservatives, for example, can help to maintain the quality of the food and reduce the health risk caused by the food going bad.

See the list of additives in our food at the end of this chapter for more discussion on the additives issue.

Although we do not yet know all the possible effects on our health of food additives, it is clear that the use of some substances becomes unhealthy when it exceeds a certain level.

Another problem is that some people suffer from allergic reactions to certain substances even if there is only a small amount in the food. The additives mentioned in Figure 2.2.10 in particular are suspected of causing or exacerbating food intolerance.

Figure 2.2.8
Additives are allowed in 'ordinary' jam but not in 'extra', 'fresh fruit' jam.

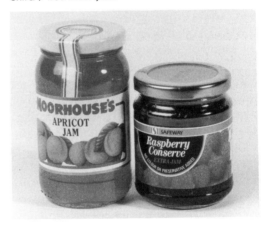

Figure : 2.2.9
Additives linked to food intolerance

Additives	E number
preservatives	E210 to E219
antioxidants	E310, E311, E312, E320, E321
azo colouring agents	E102, E124
other colouring agents	E127
flavour enhancers	620 to 625
aroma and taste enhancers	vanillin, ethylvanillin

It is estimated that some one million people in the United Kingdom suffer from intolerance to additives. The most common symptoms are itching, urticaria, fatigue, headaches, a general feeling of discomfort and pain in the joints. The quantity of additives in your diet can be reduced by having a varied diet, and particularly by choosing as many fresh, unprocessed products as possible.

The Food and Safety Act (1991) sets down requirements for the quality of food. It stipulates that foodstuffs must not be harmful to public health and that they must be traded honestly which means, for example, that milk may not be watered down. The Food and Safety Act also states which colouring agents may be added (all others being prohibited), the standards which food products must meet and the ingredients they may contain if they are to be described by certain names. However, the statute can be circumvented by using imaginative names. According to the Food and Safety Act, products such as meat, fish and chicken may not be combined with vegetable protein but there is no such regulation if names such as 'hamburger', 'fishburger' or 'chickenburger' are used.

Compliance with the Food and Safety Act is monitored by Trading Standards Officers (labelling of food) and Environmental Health Officers (hygiene and microbiological contamination of food). These officers may pay unexpected visits to kitchens in restaurants, fish and chip shops, bars, shops, markets, hospitals, nursing homes and factories. They inspect the foodstuffs they find to ensure that they conform with the requirements of the Act. For example, they check that any 'best before' date has not passed and that the area is hygienic; they may evaluate the smell, taste and appearance of foodstuffs, and they can take samples for laboratory analysis.

The **'Best before'** date can be defined as the date by which the food is recommended to be eaten, otherwise the food may become unfit to eat and even become dangerous.

The **'Use by'** date is the last date that the food is legally allowed to be sold as 'fit for human consumption'. It is the final date for use of a microbiologically highly perishable food.

Study activity 5

A 'use-by' date must be stated on the packaging of products which spoil quickly, such as milk, dairy products and meat. The producer guarantees optimal quality up to that date, after which the product may no longer be sold. Have you ever found a product in the shop after the 'use-by' date had expired, or found a foreign body in a food product? What did you (or would you) do about it? Would you say nothing and select another item? Ask for a discount? Tell the store manager? Call the Environmental Health Department or Trading Standards Officer? Can you think of another alternative?

6. Packaging of foodstuffs

In the past, many foodstuffs went directly from the farmer to the market or local shops, where they were mostly sold loose or in paper bags. The shop owner would provide details about the products so that you knew what you were buying. Nowadays, most foodstuffs are pre-packed. An attractive carton or plastic bag (or both) may benefit hygiene, but it also increases our mountains of waste. Furthermore, the packaging can look so attractive that attention is diverted from the contents.

To help us to judge the quality of a packaged product, information on the label is now compulsory giving the information listed in Figure 2.2.12. Almost all food sold in the UK must comply with the Food Labelling Regulations (1984).

Figure 2.2.10
Additives

Subtraction of additives equals risk

One man's meat ... Simone Sekers wonders if we're at all ready for a preservative-free world.

... I have begun to think long and hard about the wisdom of swapping a small amount of a chemical for a large dose of salmonella. I know that there is a vociferous and powerful body of opinion which reacts badly, both physically and mentally, to such suggestions, but the fact is that preservative-free meat products present as great a risk as the preservatives themselves.

For all the asthmatics who find their condition exacerbated by sodium metabisulphite, for all the hyperactive children who might throw another tantrum after eating a hot dog seasoned with a smidgen of sodium nitrate, there could be many more, especially the babies, the old and the weak, who might actually die of a campylobacter infection.

Now I know that we should all take great care when buying and storing food, in order to compensate for the reduction of preservative additives. I know equally that a once-a-week shop is the best many of us can manage, so busy are we proving our independence through exhausting careers.

I know that means the pork pies, the beef-burgers, the sausages, the cook-chill chicken korma might have to spend longer in the stuffy car boot than is absolutely advisable, and I know that in all probability the temperature in the fridge at home (let alone that of the chilled cabinet in the shop) is going to be higher than the recommended safety level, especially just after it has been stuffed full of perishable food at car-boot temperatures.

It will take some time for that temperature to re-establish itself too, so there is ample opportunity for worrying organisms to flourish, unchecked as they often now are by taboo additives. Moreover, since the manufacturers of fridges tend to fill them full of useless gadgets such as chilled drink dispensers rather than equip them with all-important thermometers, we are not going to know when the temperature has reached its safe zone of 5°C.

The Wise Housewife will, of course, always carry an insulated bag containing an ice pack or two and immediately transfer all perishable food to that when loading the boot with her shopping. The Foolish Housewife will not have thought of such a thing and the Forgetful Housewife will have left the bag on the kitchen table, along with the shopping list. For those of us lacking in wisdom or memory, preservatives are a godsend.

... I am not for one moment suggesting that chemical preservatives should be used as a cover for slack production methods or lack of care over hygiene and safe storage, whether commercially or at home: only that, given human frailties, a frayed chain of command snapping in the kitchens of a hospital or old people's home, too few preservatives can be a bad thing.

Once upon a time a kipper was a relatively long-lived item: modern methods and modern tastes have reduced salting and smoking, so these processes tend to be cosmetic rather than preservative – I have several times bought kippers on a Thursday to find that they only just staggered through in a fit condition until Sunday breakfast.

Many people who seek out nitrite-free bacon are somewhat surprised by its saltiness – extra salt being necessary to replace the nitrites upon which modern bacon-curing depends. The reaction that occurs in the body – where nitrates change to nitrosamines, noted to cause cancer in animals – has given rise to alarm, but salt carries other risks to heart and blood pressure. Bacon low in salt or low in nitrites equals bacon which presents a risk of food poisoning, particularly if it has the high water content of much mass-produced bacon.

I would feel a great deal safer buying a warm pasty from a baker who makes his own if he didn't display so proudly over his warming cabinet the sign stating that none of his pies and pasties contained preservative. I only wish they did ...

© Simone Sekers

Figure 2.2.11
Compulsory information on packaging

1. The name of the food.
2. A list of ingredients listed in order of quantity (i.e. greatest quantity first).
3. An indication of minimum durability.
4. Any special storage conditions.
5. The weight, volume, or number in pack.
6. The name and address of the manufacturer, packer, or seller.
7. The place of origin.
8. Instructions for use (where omitting them would make it difficult to use the product properly).

An example of a typical food label (Figure 2.2.13) illustrates the above information.

Figure 2.2.12
Food label

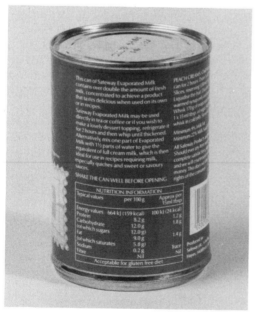

7. E numbers

All categories of additives must be listed in the ingredients. The prefix 'E' stands for European and this signifies that the additive which has been used is recognised as being safe in the countries of the European Union. In the UK, additives are approved by the Food and Safety Act (1991) and each additive is given an E number which is consistent throughout Europe. The numbers can be roughly classified as follows:

E100-E200   colouring agents;
E200-E300   preservatives and supporting substances, food acids;
E300-E400   antioxidants and/or food acids;
E400-E500   emulsifiers, stabilisers, thickening agents and/or gelling agents.

In addition, there are additives with only a number. These substances have been approved in the UK but are only provisionally allowed in the European Union as they have not yet been fully tested. There are also additives with no number, which have not been tested by the EU and include most aroma and flavour enhancers. There is a negative list of substances that are prohibited from use in the EU because they are harmful, but all other substances may be added to food as long as no harmful effects can be proven. There are thousands of these, and they are indicated with their own name or with their group name.

In Appendix 1 you will find an E number list with the names, characteristics and risks of the relevant additives. Where a small 'e' appears on the packaging, it indicates that the weight or quantity stated is an average, and the actual weight or quantity may be slightly over or under the figure given.

8. Claims

The Food Labelling Regulations make provision for certain claims on labels. They do not state precisely what could constitute a claim and a statement of the energy content of a food does not constitute a claim. However, a special schedule in the regulations specified the criteria which must be met if certain words or descriptions are to be used. Examples of these are the criteria for use of the words 'dietary' or 'dietetic'.

These may be applied to food which 'has been specially made for people whose digestive process or metabolism is disturbed or who, by reason of their special physiological condition, obtain special benefit from a controlled consumption of certain substances.'

Diabetic Claims
The food must normally be higher in fat or energy than similar 'non-diabetic' foods and it must not contain more mono- or disaccharide than is necessary. If a diabetic food contains fructose, sorbitol, mannitol, xylitol, isomalt, or hydrogenated glucose syrup, the label must make the recommendation that a total of no more than 25g of these substances should be eaten daily.

'Light' Foods
There is currently proposed a European directive on the use of some claims on packaging. In particular, the use of the word 'light' is currently being scrutinised. This term refers to a food product that has significantly less energy than the regular or ordinary product. Food products with labels carrying the word are likely to contain 25% less energy than a similar product. Thus the food will contain less fat and/or sugar. Similarly, foods labelled as high or rich in a particular nutrient are likely to contain 50% more than un-supplemented items in the new directive. Specific health claims are to be investigated by the Department of Health this year.

Slimming Claims
Slimming claims may only be made if the food is 'capable of contributing to weight loss.' If a food is claimed to be 'reduced energy' it must have an energy value of no more than 75% compared with the same weight of an equivalent food which does not carry a claim. To qualify for a 'low energy' claim a food must contain no more than 167kJ (40kcal)/100g or 100ml and the energy value of a normal portion must be no more than 167kJ (40kcal).

Study activity 6
a. Why should the name and address of the producer be given on packaging?
b. Look at the packaging of a food product. Is all the required information actually stated? Are the meanings all clear? Is this product in the food guide? If so, where? Is the price of the product in proportion to its nutritional value?
c. Collect food labels or packaging. Divide them into two groups: those which state that additives have been added and those which do not.
d. What is your own opinion about the use of additives in foodstuffs?

9. Summary

Informational models may be useful tools for evaluating a diet and for planning a healthy diet. In this chapter, we discussed the purpose and use of food guides. We have discussed how the Canadian model in particular was created, what the underlying principles are, how foodstuffs are classified, and what guidelines to follow.

We also looked at the issue of additives in food. These substances may be used for a variety of reasons and have advantages and disadvantages. The Government has some influence on the quality of foodstuffs through such instruments as the Food and Safety Act and Trading Standards Commission. Compliance with this statute is monitored by the Environmental Health Department.

The Government is advised on aspects of food safety and food composition by a statutory body (Food Advisory Committee). Labelling regulations make it compulsory to give a certain amount of data on the packaging. The meaning of some of the terminology used on labels has been explained in some detail, and we have seen how this can provide useful information for evaluating the quality of a food product. The chapter also contains an overview of the recommended amounts of food required to formulate a healthy diet containing the correct quantities of nutrients.

Figure 2.2.13
Additives in our food

Group Name	Effect	Found in
anti-caking agents	prevent lumps forming in powdered foodstuffs in their containers	icing sugar, dried salt, powdered milk
antioxidants	protect against deterioration due to oxygen in the air	salad dressing, mayonnaise, beer, biscuits
anti-foaming agents	prevent foaming during production	soup, jam
preservatives	prevent spoilage from bacteria and mould, i.e. extend the shelf life	wine, beer, tinned potatoes, jam, lemonade, meat products, soup, mayonnaise, margarine, salad dressing
emulsifiers	enable fat and water to be mixed together	mayonnaise, salad dressing, margarine
gelling agents	thickening agents to make fruit products firmer	jam, desserts, fruit products
aroma and flavour enhancers	add a specific aroma or flavour	sweets, lemonade, desserts, fruit yoghurt, sausages, custard
glazing agents	provide a shiny layer, usually a thin wax-like coating	raisins, some sweets
colouring agents	used to colour foodstuffs	strawberry jam, fruit yoghurt, sweets, margarine, custard, fruit loaf, beer
artificial sweeteners	add a sweet flavour without adding energy	beer, soft drinks, products for diabetics

Group Name	Effect	Found in
flour enhancers	provide a more even crumb spread in bread	flour for bread
raising agents	make dough rise without yeast	self-raising flour, biscuits, cakes
flavour enhancers	enhance the flavour	tinned soup, dried soup, sauces, sausages, various snacks
melting salts	allow cheese to melt without the fat running out	soft cheese, spreading cheese
stabilisers	stabilise the form of the product (by, for example, preventing the leakage of water from meat products, or the separation of particles in liquid products)	mayonnaise, salad dressing, meat products, ice cream, flavoured milk
thickening agents	thicken the product	puddings, ice cream, salad dressing, low fat margarine
food acids	acids which are used to pickle foodstuffs, or to increase the sour taste	jam, fruit juice, salad dressing, sour pickles, sour dairy products
acidity regulators	adjust the degree of sourness in the taste	ice cream, dairy products with fruit juice, meat products

The nutrients

1. Introduction

In this chapter we will examine the substances in food which are essential for the human body. These are known as nutrients. We will investigate precisely what we consume, and the effect this has on our health. Before exploring this, however, we will discuss how food is digested, absorbed, and used. In addition, we will take a look at how we are provided with energy and the function it has in the body.

Learning outcomes

After studying this chapter the student should be able to:
- describe in her own words what digestion means;
- describe how protein, fats and carbohydrates are digested and in what form they are absorbed by the body;
- give two reasons why human beings need energy every day;
- name four different factors affecting a person's energy requirement;
- state which substances in food provide energy, and how much energy they each provide per gram;
- calculate how many grams of protein a person needs per day;
- indicate how much water a person needs per day, why it is needed, and in what ways it can be absorbed;
- explain the functions of carbohydrates, fats, protein, water, vitamins, and minerals;
- divide carbohydrates and fats each into six types, protein into two types, then list three examples of foodstuffs for each of these groups;
- explain why dietary fibre has a positive effect on intestinal function;
- explain why it is recommended to consume fat in moderation, but to eat plenty of starch and complex carbohydrates;
- name some foodstuffs which are rich in protein, carbohydrates and fat and list five foodstuffs for each of these three groups;
- describe the symptoms of dehydration;
- describe the situations in which it would be useful to keep a fluid balance chart;
- explain what cholesterol is, in which foodstuffs it can be found, and the possible effect of a high cholesterol level in the blood;

– state in which sections of the food guide each of the following nutrients appear: iron, calcium, vitamins A, B1, B2, B6, B12, folic acid, vitamins C, D, E and K.

Figure 2.3.1
The digestive tract

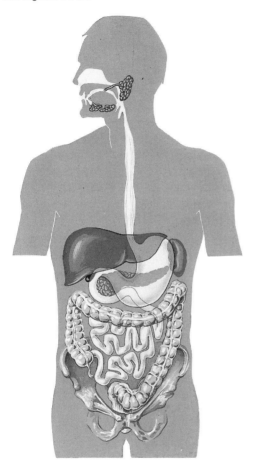

the colon and is eliminated. The digestive tract, and the digestive processes which take place, are described in Figure 2.3.2.

The nutrients in food are broken down by digestive juices into smaller units: proteins into amino acids, fats into fatty acids and glycerol, and carbohydrates into simple sugars. In these forms, nutrients pass through the intestine, allowing them to be absorbed into the bloodstream.

Vitamins and minerals occur in food as micronutrients. They can pass through the intestinal lining without the aid of digestive juices. Optimal digestion is effected by adequate dentition, tongue and swallowing functions. Fats can only be properly digested in combination with bile, which emulsifies fats – that is, it divides fat into small globules so that it can be efficiently broken down by the pancreatic enzymes and gastric juices.

Study activity 1

a. You eat a slice of brown bread with butter and cheese. Brown bread contains, among other things, starch, iron and vitamin B. Cheese provides a lot of calcium and protein. Butter contains fat, vitamin A and vitamin D. What happens to this sandwich in the digestive system and which substances ultimately end up in the bloodstream?

b. Why is it more healthy to chew slowly?

2. The digestive system

The nutrients present in our food are made available to the body by the digestive system (Figure 2.3.1). During the digestion process, the nutrients are broken down to such an extent that they can be absorbed by blood and lymphatic vessels through the intestinal wall. The indigestible and undigested food residue passes through

3. Energy

Everything a person does requires energy. This is true for both external effort (such as walking, cycling, reading, writing and standing) and internal effort (such as breathing, digesting food, functioning of the heart and maintaining body temperature). This means that we use energy even when we are sleeping or resting.

Figure 2.3.2
Digestive processes

Section of digestive tract	Digestive gland	Digestive juices produced (active agents)	Nutrient which is processed	Absorption of nutrients
mouth	salivary gland	saliva (amylase)	starch	none
stomach	gastric juice glands	gastric juice (pepsin, hydrochloric acid)	proteins	none
duodenum	pancreas	pancreatic juice (trypsin, amylase, lipase)	proteins, starch, fats	water, minerals
	liver	bile (bile salts)	fats	none
small intestine (jejunum, ileum)	intestinal juice glands	intestinal juice (lipase, erepsin)	protein blocks, fats	amino acids, fatty acids + glycerol
		(maltase, lactase, sucrase)	carbohydrates (maltose, lactose, sucrose)	simple carbohydrates (e.g. glucose)
				water, vitamins, minerals
large intestine (colon)		bacteria flora		water, vitamins, minerals

a. Requirement

The amount of energy a person needs per day depends on a variety of factors:
- age
- gender
- height and build
- amount of physical activity.

Figure 2.3.3 gives a guide to the average amount of energy you need per day. By international agreement, energy is expressed in joules. Before 1978, the unit commonly used was the kilocalorie (kcal), but in dietetics this has now been largely replaced by kJ (1 kcal = 4.2 kJ). 1 megajoule

Figure 2.3. 3
Energy requirement for
moderate exertion*

Age Group	Women weight (in kg)	Women requirement (in MJ)	Men weight (in kg)	Men requirement (in MJ)
16-20 yrs	58	9.7	66	13.4
20-35 yrs	60	9.2	70	12.2
35-55 yrs	60	8.8	70	11.3
55-75 yrs	60	8.4	68	10.5
> 75 yrs	60	7.1	65	8.4

* Moderate exertion is approximately 6-8 hours of sitting activities and 1-2 hours of fairly intensive exertion in a 24-hour period.

(MJ) = 1,000 kilojoules. In the United Kingdom, however, kilocalorie is still widely used in slimming magazines, advertisements, popular weight-reducing diets and food labelling.

If a person absorbs as much energy from his food as he uses, his body weight will remain the same. Provided that the body is not retaining fluid, body weight is the best way to monitor the balance between energy absorption and energy consumption.

As age increases, the energy requirement decreases even if the amount of physical exercise remains the same. Older people have a lower metabolic rate than younger people because the body's cellular activity reduces as one gets older. A man of 65 will require 15% less energy than a 25-year-old carrying out the same physical activity. Thus, if he absorbs the same amount of energy, the surplus energy will be stored in the body and the body weight will increase. The consequences of obesity will be discussed in Module 3, Chapter 4.

Figure 2.3.3 also shows that the energy requirements differ between men and women. Men need more energy because their relatively greater muscle mass results in a higher metabolic rate. Figure 2.3.4 shows how increased physical exertion requires more energy.

Figure 2.3.4
Energy requirements for different activities

A young woman weighing 60 kg uses, per minute:

sleeping, lying down	4 kJ
sitting quietly	5 kJ
standing	6 kJ
eating/drinking	6 kJ
writing	6 kJ
getting dressed	10 kJ
washing	11 kJ
driving a car	12 kJ
washing the dishes	13 kJ
walking at 2.5 miles/hr (4 km/hr)	15 kJ
making the bed	16 kJ
having a shower	17 kJ
swimming	21 kJ
dancing	23 kJ
playing tennis	30 kJ
climbing stairs	35 kJ
lifting heavy objects (5 kg)	39 kJ
skiing	42 kJ
cycling at 20 km/hour	46 kJ
running at 15 km/hour	55 kJ

Study activity 2

Susan is a nurse who works in a large city hospital. This morning she took 25 minutes to drive to work. She had to walk for five minutes to reach her ward. During her duties that morning she spent approximately 1 hour walking and half an hour standing talking to the patients. During her coffee break and the staff meeting, she sat quietly for 45 minutes. Then she spent half an hour making beds and 15 minutes lifting patients (helping them from chairs, to the toilets, etc.). Calculate the amount of energy she expended and therefore needed over these four hours.

The amount of energy Susan used in these four hours is equal to the energy from:
4 slices of brown bread and butter with 2 slices of cheese and 1 tomato
or:
1 bag of chips with ketchup, 1 sausage, 1 glass of apple juice.

b. What substances in food provide energy?
The greater part of the energy derived from food comes from carbohydrates, but fats are also an important source of energy. Proteins can also serve as fuel to some degree, and although not a nutrient, alcohol does provide energy. The amount of energy that these substances provide is as follows:

1 gram of carbohydrates	17 kJ
1 gram of fat	38 kJ
1 gram of protein	17 kJ
1 gram of alcohol	29 kJ

4. Carbohydrates

Carbohydrates are organic compounds including sugars, polysaccharides and starch, which contain carbon, hydrogen and oxygen. They constitute an important source of food for all animals. Carbohydrates have an important place in our daily diet. In a healthy diet, they provide 50-55% of the energy (Figure 2.3.5).

a. Functions of carbohydrates
Carbohydrates are an important source of energy with one gram of carbohydrates providing 17 kJ. Limited reserves of carbohydrates can be formed in the liver and

muscles in the form of glycogen. However, surplus carbohydrate in the diet is converted into fat. The indigestible carbohydrates are useful for bowel motility and function.

Figure 2.3.5
More than half of our daily energy is provided by carbohydrates:

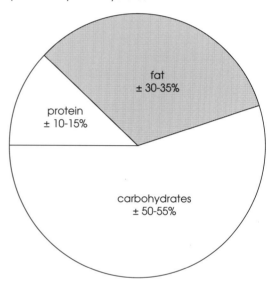

b. Carbohydrates in our food
Carbohydrates are found particularly in foods of vegetable origin. We can divide the carbohydrates into two categories:

–   ***The digestible carbohydrates***
    These include simple and complex carbohydrates and starch. Amongst the simple carbohydrates, glucose is widely found, and fructose (or fruit sugar) is found in fruit. The complex carbohydrates include sucrose which is found in ordinary table sugar or honey and in foodstuffs which contain these products, such as sweets, biscuits, soft drinks, jam and concentrated fruit squash. Lactose (milk sugar) is also found naturally in milk and other dairy products.
    Starch is found in wheat, rye, oats, barley, rice, potatoes, bread, macaroni,

spaghetti, wheat flour and cornflour. It is a common belief that granulated sugar is necessary for providing the muscles with energy. However, all digestible carbohydrates are important energy-providers and supply fuel for muscular effort, amongst other things. They are broken down in the digestive tract and ultimately end up in the bloodstream in the form of glucose, galactose or fructose. Galactose and fructose are converted into glucose in the liver. The glucose is then transported through the bloodstream to the body's cells where it is burned, thus releasing its energy.

It is now known that sugar, and foodstuffs containing sugar, can affect the teeth by contributing to dental caries (Figure 2.3.6). Bacteria in the mouth convert sugar into acid which attacks the tooth's enamel. In order to prevent tooth decay, it is recommended that we do not eat sugar on more than six or seven occasions per day. Eating more meals or snacks than this does not allow the teeth sufficient time to recover from the acid attack.

– *The indigestible carbohydrates (dietary fibre).*
Dietary fibre cannot be digested but it does perform a useful function in the body in that it provides faecal bulk. It is found in wholemeal cereal products (such as wholemeal bread and unpolished rice), vegetables, fruit, potatoes, pulses and nuts. The outer layer of a cereal grain, in particular, contains a great deal of dietary fibre. A well-known example is bran, which is the outer layer of a wheat grain.

Unfortunately, these important substances have disappeared from the diets of many people. People often choose a refined diet which contains white bread, white rice, biscuits and flour. These products contain very little dietary fibre and far fewer vitamins and minerals than, for instance, wholemeal bread, unpolished rice and wholemeal biscuits.

Dietary fibre attracts liquid, which makes the faeces softer and bulkier, and it is passed through the colon comparatively quickly. In addition, dietary fibre assists the chewing process. You must chew longer on a piece of wholemeal bread than on a piece of white bread, and this has a positive effect on your teeth and gives you a feeling of fullness.

By examining levels of dietary fibre, starch, sugars, vitamins and minerals, we can assess the quality of different food products. Figure 2.3.8 gives examples of this.

Figure 2.3.6
A lot of teeth are lost to dental caries.

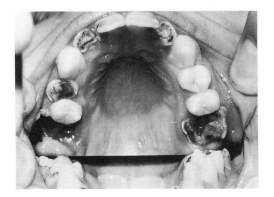

Figure 2.3.7
Foods which contain carbohydrates

Food	Preferred choice	Acceptable	To be avoided
bread	wholemeal varieties, wholewheat crispbread, ryebread	white bread, fruit loaf, cream cracker	croissant
breakfast foods	porridge, muesli, oatmeal, bran flakes	cornflakes and other cereals	
potatoes	boiled potatoes	mashed potatoes, roast potatoes (vegetable oil)	fried potatoes, chips (cooked in animal fat)
pulses, legumes	beans and peas, tinned sweet corn, lentils		
rice, pasta	unpolished brown rice, wholemeal pasta	macaroni and spaghetti	
vegetables	boiled, baked, raw	vegetables in a thick sauce (creamed), raw vegetables with dip	fried vegetables (cooked in animal fat)
fruit	all types of fresh fruit in its own juice in a jar or tin	fruit in syrup, orange juice, grapefruit juice, dried fruit, apple juice	
sweet snacks	wholemeal biscuits	Danish pastries, fruit cake, low fat ice cream	chocolate cake, cream cakes, full fat ice cream

Figure 2.3.8
Carbohydrate content (simple and complex) in some foodstuffs

cheese	0%
cabbage	4%
apple	10%
soft drinks	12%
baked beans	13%
grapes	16%
potatoes (boiled)	17%
fruit cocktail (in syrup)	20%
banana	22%
ice cream	24%
pasta	24%
tomato ketchup	25%
rice (white)	31%
wholemeal bread	44%
white bread	49%
Danish pastry	51%
crispbread	58%
chocolate	59%
shredded wheat	68%
cornflakes	84%

Study activity 3

a. What foodstuffs from the food guide provide carbohydrates? Indicate the groups or sections in which they can be found. In which groups or sections are products rich in dietary fibre found?

b. Indicate what types of carbohydrates are found in the following foods (distinguish between fructose, lactose, sucrose, starch and dietary fibre): yoghurt, wholemeal bread, white bread, apple, orange, bran, spinach, lentils, porridge, oatmeal, lemonade, cake.

c. Explain why starch and dietary fibre should be an important constituent in a balanced diet.

d. Why is an apple a healthier snack than a bar of chocolate? Why is wholemeal bread healthier than white bread?

e. How much carbohydrate do the following contain:
one slice of bread, one apple, 1 tub (150 ml) of low fat yoghurt, 1 glass (150 ml) of a soft drink?

f. Check how much granulated sugar you add to coffee, tea or other drinks and meals every day.

Figure 2.3.9
The amount of sugar in cakes and soft drinks

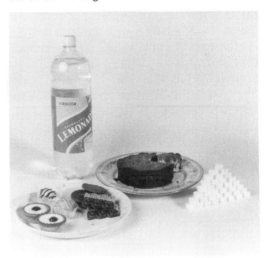

5. Fats

Fats are soft solids found in some plants and in animal tissue

a. Functions of fats
Fats provide energy (38 kJ per gram). A reserve of fat can be created in the body and this may be useful when someone is ill or suffering from a temporary loss of appetite. The fat beneath the skin helps to insulate the body and the fat surrounding organs such as the kidneys has a protective function.

Fats can carry those vitamins which are soluble in fat, such as vitamins A and D. A diet with an exceptionally low fat content can, therefore, lead to a deficiency in vitamins A and D.

b. Requirement

Like carbohydrates, fats are an important source of energy and they should supply approximately 33% of our total energy requirement. On average, however, fat consumption is too high (at around 40% of our total energy intake). Around half of current fat consumption is in the form of 'visible' fat (or obvious, easily seen) such as butter, margarine, oil, cooking fat, whipped cream and mayonnaise which consist almost entirely of fat. The rest, however, comes from foodstuffs with an 'invisible' fat content, where the fat is highly emulsified and therefore not recognised as a major fat source. Such food items include full fat cheese, full fat dairy products, nuts, crisps, biscuits, pastry, sausages, pâté, fatty fish (such as mackerel, salmon, herring) and ice cream (Figure 2.3.10).

Figure 2.3.10
Invisible fats

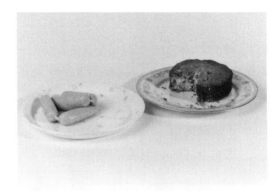

Figure 2.3.11
Food and Your Heart, British Heart Foundation, 1992 London

What is a saturated fat?

The basic building blocks which go to make up the fat in foods are called *fatty acids* and depending on their chemical structure they can be described as either saturated or unsaturated. The difference between one fat or oil and another will depend on whether it contains a lot of saturated or unsaturated fatty acids. A food which is described as "high in saturated fat" is *mostly* built up from saturated fatty acid units. Fats like lard and butter, which are solid at room temperature contain a lot of saturated fatty acids. More saturated fats are found in animal foods like meat and in dairy products. Chicken, turkey, rabbit and oily fish, like herring, have fats which are less saturated than other animal fats.

The other type of building block, the unsaturated fatty acids, can vary between the most unsaturated (polyunsaturated) and least unsaturated (mono-unsaturated), When people talk about a fat being "high in polyunsaturates" it is one where there are more polyunsaturated fatty acids than saturated ones. Oils, which are liquid at room temperature, usually have a high level of polyunsaturated fatty acids. *Margarine is made by taking oils and changing some of the unsaturated fatty acids into saturated ones – making a solid product. Some margarines contain just as much saturated fat as butter. But a soft margarine is more likely to contain higher levels of polyunsaturates.

*Fats from plant sources, like nuts, are generally less saturated but two plant oils, coconut and palm oil, are highly saturated.

The chart below shows the foods that are higher and lower in saturated fat. (*shows that the food is lower in total fat).

Foods higher in saturated fat	Foods lower in saturated fat
Butter, lard, most margarines	Margarines "high in polyunsaturates", low fat spreads*
"Cooking oil" (unspecified) is usually high in saturated fats (coconut oil, palm oil)	Corn (maize) oil, sun-flower oil, safflower oil, olive oil
Lamb, pork, beef	Fish*. chicken*, turkey
Cheeses like Cheddar	Edam*, Brie*, cottage cheese*, fromage frais
Whole milk, cream	Skimmed*, semi-skimmed milk*

c. The fats in our food

The fats found in our food (Figure 2.3.12) can be classified in two ways

- **According to origin:**
  vegetable origin (e.g., sunflower oil, olive oil, nuts, vegetable margarine, cocoa fat, coconut fat)
  animal origin (e.g., butter, full fat milk, cheese, bacon, sausages)
- **According to composition:**
  unsaturated fats – These fats are predominantly found in liquid or soft fat forms, such as corn oil, sunflower oil, olive oil, nuts, peanut butter, low fat margarine (60-65% linoleic acid), vegetable (tub) margarine (40% or more linoleic acid), salad dressing, mayonnaise and fatty fish. The unsaturated fats can play an important role in preventing heart and arterial disease, as they can actually reduce the cholesterol level in the blood. The unsaturated fats can be classified as monounsaturated or polyunsaturated. Monounsaturated fats (containing one double bond in their chemical structure), such as oleic acid, are widely found in certain foods like olive oil, avocado pears, and fatty fish. Polyunsaturates (containing more than one double bond in their chemical structure), such as linoleic acid, are found in vegetable seed oils like corn oil, sunflower oil, and rapeseed.
  saturated fats – These acids, such as palmitic and stearic acids, contain only one single bond in their chemical structure and are found particularly in hard fats and animal fats, such as packet margarine, butter, full fat milk, cheese, fatty meat, chocolate, whipped cream, many types of pastries, biscuits, cooking fat, deep-frying fat (and thus the products which are fried in it), coconut oil, and powdered whole milk. Saturated fats can raise the cholesterol level in the blood, thereby increasing the risk of heart and arterial disease.

Figure 2.3.12
Fat content of some foodstuffs

vegetable oil	100%
butter	82%
margarine	82%
mayonnaise	76%
peanuts	47%
low fat margarine	41%
crisps	37%
Cheddar cheese (full fat)	34%
chocolate	30%
corned beef	27%
luncheon meat	27%
cake	26%
pork sausage (grilled)	25%
Edam cheese	25%
digestive biscuits	21%
chips	16%
pâté	15%
minced beef	15%
lean pork chop	11%
mackerel	11%
ham	6%
wholemilk	4%
full fat yoghurt	3%
semi-skimmed milk	2%
cornflakes	1%
low fat yoghurt	1%
rice	1%
pasta	1%
potatoes	0%

d. The role of cholesterol

Cholesterol is a fatty substance which is only found in animal foodstuffs. The human body can also produce cholesterol internally - it is an essential substance in the body, used as a precursor of vitamin D, hormones, and nerve tissue. However, a high cholesterol concentration in the blood increases the risk of heart and arterial disease. Because of this, cholesterol in food has been unfairly maligned. Most of the cholesterol in the body is produced internally, and the amount of cholesterol in food has only a slight influence on the cholesterol level in the blood. The total level of saturated fats in the diet has a far greater influence on the cholesterol concentration in the blood than the cholesterol content of the diet on its own. Foodstuffs with a high cholesterol content include egg yolk, liver, kidneys, shellfish, butter and cream.

Figure 2.3.13
The Flora Project for Heart Disease Prevention, London

What choices can I make?

The next time you reach for an item on the supermarket shelf – STOP- and check the label – ingredients are listed in order of quantities. Ask yourself "Is this a healthier alternative to what I normally buy?" – Try to buy foods high in polyunsaturates or high in fibre, particularly soluble fibre – watch out for those high in fat, especially saturated fat, sugar or salt.

Choose these:

1. Cottage cheese, low fat cheese or cheese alternatives which are made with sunflower oil
2. Skimmed or semi-skimmed milk, low fat natural yoghurt or low fat fromage frais
3. Sunflower margarine, low fat spreads, oils and fats which are high in polyunsaturates
4. Lean meat, poultry and fish
5. Grilled, poached or steamed foods
6. High fibre wholegrain varieties of bread, breakfast cereals, rice, oats, pasta, beans and pulses
7. Fresh vegetables, fruit or canned fruit in natural juices
8. Mayonnaise alternatives and salad dressings which are high in polyunsaturates or low in fat

In preference to these:

1. Cheddar cheese, Stilton and other full fat cheeses
2. Whole milk and cream
3. Butter, hard margarine and fats, lard or suet
4. Fatty meat and meat products (pies, sausages, pâtés)
5. Fried foods
6. White bread and pre-sweetened breakfast cereals
7. Canned fruit in syrup, cakes, biscuits and sweets
8. Traditional mayonnaise and oily salad dressings which are not high in polyunsaturates

Food for Thought

The traditional British diet has surrendered! After years of attack by health professionals in magazines, newspapers, books and TV programmes – old eating habits are finally being swept away. It's now clearly understood that good diet is linked to good health.

Eating a poor diet has been linked to a battery of illnesses. Obesity, heart disease, digestive problems, even some cancers can all follow bad eating habits. But ill health doesn't happen overnight. It can take many years to develop, often with no outward signs. But the good news is that changing to a healthier diet and lifestyle can help prevent these, and many other diseases.

And opting for a healthy diet need not be hard work, a few simple changes can soon put you on the right road:

– Reduce the total amount of fat you eat especially saturated fats and partially replace with polyunsaturated fats. Eat more fresh fish, lean meat and poultry, rather than high saturated fat foods such as sausages and burgers.
– Increase your intake of fibre-rich starchy foods, such as wholemeal bread and pasta, baked jacket potatoes, high fibre breakfast cereals, oats and pulses.
– Eat plenty of fresh fruit and vegetables.
– Cut down your sugar by opting for unsweetened fruit juices or low calorie soft drinks and eating less sugary foods such as cakes, puddings, sweets and biscuits.
– Limit the quantity of salt you take by using less in cooking and at the table and by eating fresh fruit instead of salty crisps and nuts – which are also high in fat.

e. Feeling hungry and fats in the diet
The digestion of fat in food takes far longer than the digestion of carbohydrates and protein. This is because fat slows down the passage of food through the stomach, so that a meal rich in fat will remain in the stomach longer. This is known as the satiety value of fat. As a result, you will feel full for a longer period of time after eating a meal with a lot of gravy and fatty meat than after eating a meal without much fat. This partly explains why people trying to lose weight, and who consequently eat less fat, complain of intense hunger. Using the type and amount of fat as a basis, we can divide foods into degrees of preference (Figure 2.3.14).

Study activity 4

  a. What sections of the food guide include foodstuffs containing fat?
  b. Why is it recommended that you consume saturated fat in moderation?
  c. What are the differences and similarities between butter and soft margarine?
  d. What is the difference between margarine and low fat margarine?
  e. Name three foodstuffs which can raise the concentration of cholesterol in the blood and three foodstuffs which can reduce it.
  f. Which foodstuffs containing invisible fats do you eat regularly?
  g. Write down all the products containing fat that you ate yesterday and put them into a table of three categories as in Figure 2.3.14.

6. Proteins

a. Functions of proteins
Proteins are important building substances for the body. They are present in hormones, enzymes, antibodies, and all cells, such as muscle cells, blood cells and skin cells. A process of building up and breaking down is continually taking place in the cells of the body, and we therefore need a daily intake of protein from our diet.

Proteins can also be used as a fuelling substance. If there is more protein in the diet than is necessary for building, growth or recovery, the surplus protein is burned. Each gram of protein provides 17 kJ. A high protein level in the diet will not, therefore, lead to accelerated growth or muscle development, but it may eventually stress the kidneys, which have to work extra hard to process and dispose of protein end-products.

When there is a long-term deficiency of proteins we will see, in the first instance, stunted growth, slow healing of wounds and anaemia. Feelings of fatigue and muscle weakness may occur. A person suffering from protein deficiency will become more susceptible to infections, decubitus will occur more easily and liquid may be retained in the tissues (oedema). Children will suffer from retarded growth, and have thin arms and legs and a noticeably fat stomach due to liquid retention. Protein deficiency occurs particularly among alcoholics, patients who have undergone major surgery and people with burns or cancer.

b. Requirement
Ten to fifteen per cent of the energy which is needed in a balanced diet should be provided by protein. The protein requirement depends on, amongst other things, the body weight. Under normal circumstances a person has a daily requirement of approximately 0.75 grams of protein per kilogram of ideal body weight. For example, someone with a normal body weight of 60 kg needs 60 x 0.75 = 45 grams of protein per day. This is more than adequately covered by the average UK intake of 70-80 grams of protein per person per day. Protein requirement is higher in certain situations, including when the body is still growing, in women who are pregnant or breast-feeding, during illness and recovery (such as after surgery when there may be wounds, serious blood loss and burn injury) and for athletes in training.

Figure 2.3.14
Foods which contain fat

Food	Preferred choice	Acceptable	To be avoided
milk and other dairy products	skimmed milk, very low fat yoghurt, buttermilk	semi-skimmed milk, low fat yoghurt	full fat milk, full fat yoghurt, full cream, sour cream
cheese	cottage cheese, low fat cheese, low fat spreading cheese, fromage frais	medium fat cheese	Stilton, Cheddar, all full fat cheeses
meat products	roast beef, turkey, ham, chicken, shoulder ham	rib of beef, sausage meat, liver, kidney	bacon, black pudding, pâté, salami, corned beef
meat	steak, roast beef, lean beef, lean stewing steak, pork steak, loin chops	minced beef, spare ribs	belly pork, any fatty meats
chicken, turkey	turkey fillet, chicken fillet		chicken with skin
eggs		scrambled, poached, boiled, no more than 3 eggs a week	omelettes, fried eggs
fish, shellfish	grilled, baked or boiled cod, haddock, plaice, sole, whiting, trout, salmon, mussels, tinned tuna in brine	fried trout, fried haddock, tinned salmon, steamed mackerel, herring, tinned sardines, fish fingers, kippers, smoked fish	eel, cod roe, tinned fish in various oils and sauces
on bread	low fat margarine	margarine with more than 40% unsaturated fat, medium fat butter	butter and packet margarine
cooking fat	vegetable oils	tub margarine	butter, cooking fat, ghee

Food	Preferred choice	Acceptable	To be avoided
salad dressing, sauces	tomato ketchup, salad dressing with less than 5% oil, soy sauce	salad dressing with less than 25% oil, medium fat mayonnaise	mayonnaise, salad dressing with more than 25% oil
snacks, nuts, savouries	spring rolls, pickled vegetable salad, crackers with low fat cheese, Japanese rice crackers	pizza, potato salad, sunflower seeds, fruit and nut mix, dried fruits	sausage rolls, hamburgers, crisps, peanuts, hazelnuts, walnuts

Figure 2.3.15
Protein content of some foodstuffs

lean pork	32%
bacon	30%
corned beef	27%
Cheddar cheese (full fat)	26%
Edam cheese	25%
peanuts	25%
haddock	23%
minced beef	23%
pork sausages	13%
eggs (boiled)	13%
lentils	9%
brown bread	8%
cornflakes	8%
baked beans	5%
yoghurt	4%
rice	3%
milk	3%
potatoes	2%
apple	1%
cabbage	1%

c. Proteins in our food

Most foodstuffs contain protein. The amount can vary substantially: vegetables and fruit, for example, contain very little protein, while meat, fish, cheese, milk and pulses are very rich in protein (Figure 2.3.15). In the UK, it is primarily animal proteins which are consumed, particularly in the form of meat, fish, cheese, meat products and eggs.

It is a common misconception that proteins of vegetable origin are inferior to those of animal origin. Vegetarians used to be advised to always combine different vegetable proteins, such as cereals with pulses and legumes (like pea soup with pancakes, or rice with lentils) or cereals with dairy products (such as bread and cheese). Research has shown, however, that there is no need to worry about combining proteins – at least, not for vegetarians who consume milk, cheese and eggs and who obtain sufficient energy from their diet. This is because in the UK we have sufficient variation in our diet and take in such an abundance of protein that it is almost impossible to suffer from a lack of it. A proper combination of vegetable proteins is only important for vegans, who avoid not only meat but also milk, cheese and eggs (see Module 4, Chapter 1).

Study activity 5

a. How much protein does a person need per day? How much protein is taken in daily per person in the UK?

b. Why do we need protein every day? What products rich in protein do you consume regularly?

c. Can a person live without animal protein?

d. What foodstuffs from the food guide contain a lot of protein? In which sections are they found?

e. How does a diet with sufficient protein contribute to effective resistance against disease?

f. Give two examples of meals without meat or fish which conform with the principles of the food guide.

g. Why do athletes have an increased protein requirement during the initial phase of their training?

h. Assess your protein intake and comment on its adequacy.

7. Water

a. Functions of water

With 60-65% of body weight made up of water, it is an important building substance. It is also a solvent and acts as a conveyor of substances like nutrients and residue products. With the help of water these can enter and leave cells and travel through the bloodstream and the body. Water is also important for temperature regulation, enabling the process of perspiration to cool the skin and thus helping to maintain a constant body temperature of approximately 37°C.

Figure 2.3.16
In this diagram of fluid balance the small glasses represent the external intake and loss of fluid, as well as the water production by metabolic processes in body cells. The larger glasses represent the greater volumes of fluid secreted in the intestines, but reabsorbed lower in the intestines in normal conditions. The numbers in the diagram represent volumes in litres. The total intake volume, however, may be subject to considerable variation depending on the composition of daily food (consider the volumes of beer drunk socially in a relatively short period of time by some individuals).

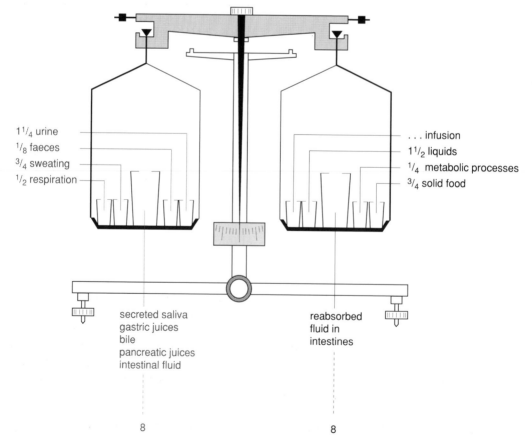

$1^1/_4$ urine
$^1/_8$ faeces
$^3/_4$ sweating
$^1/_2$ respiration

. . . infusion
$1^1/_2$ liquids
$^1/_4$ metabolic processes
$^3/_4$ solid food

secreted saliva
gastric juices
bile
pancreatic juices
intestinal fluid

reabsorbed
fluid in
intestines

8

8

Figure 2.3.17
Fluid balance chart of an adult

Fluid output		Fluid input	
urine	1000-1600 ml	drink	1000-1500 ml
perspiration	500-700 ml	food	600-900 ml
breathing	400 ml	oxidation water	400 ml
faeces	80-100 ml		
	2000-2800 ml		2000-2800 ml

b. Requirement
A human body consists of 60-65% water. If, for example, you weigh 60 kg, your body contains around 38 litres of water. Every day we lose substantial amounts of fluid in urine, perspiration, breathing and faeces, and this lost fluid must be replaced with drinks and water from food. (Figure 2.3.16) On average, a human being needs 2.5 litres of fluid daily. A fluid balance chart indicates the relationship between input and output (Figure 2.3.17).

If the fluid in the body falls below a critical level, a feeling of thirst develops. If a person takes in less than one litre of fluid per day from food and drink then dehydration occurs. Symptoms of minor dehydration include drowsiness, listlessness, lack of appetite and fatigue. Serious dehydration is characterised by dry, inelastic, loose skin and sunken eyes. A fluid loss of 20% can be fatal.

c. Fluid in our foods
We obtain our fluids from food as well as drink. Potatoes, for instance, consist of 77% water, vegetables and fruit 49% and bread 40%. We take in some 600-900 ml of liquid from food per day. The sixth recommendation for a balanced diet (see Module 2 Chapter 2) states we should have a fluid intake of at least one and a half litres every day, and alcohol should be consumed sparingly. Figure 2.3.18 shows how this fluid intake might typically be made up, and Figure 2.3.19 gives an overview of suitable and less suitable drinks.

Figure 2.3.18
Example of fluid intake from drinking 1.5 litres per day

2 cups of coffee	250 ml
4 cups of tea	500 ml
2 glasses of water	300 ml
1 glass of fruit juice	150 ml
1 glass of milk	150 ml
1 carton of yoghurt	150 ml
Total	1,500 ml

Figure 2.3.19
Choice of foods

Preferred	In moderation
tap water, mineral water, low calorie soft drinks, coffee and tea without sugar	soft drinks, squash, coffee and tea with sugar, fruit juice, beer, wine, sherry

d. Dehydration
Dehydration may occur because of:
drinking too little
This often occurs with elderly people, who may simply feel less thirsty or who may be afraid of incontinence, or of having to urinate too often or during the night. In particular, patients who cannot indicate that they are thirsty require extra attention. This might

Figure 2.3.20
Fluid balance chart

.... HOSPITAL 24 HOUR FLUID BALANCE CHART DATE						Surname First Name Unit No. Ward					
Previous 24 Hour Intake:-						Output:-		Balance:-			
Oral Intake			Intravenous Intake			Output					
Time	Nature	Vol	Time	Nature	Line 1 Vol	Line 2 Vol	Time	Urine	Gastric	1 Drain	2 Drain	Use as required

include elderly people suffering from dementia, the mentally ill, people with physical or mental disabilities, the very ill, small children, people who have swallowing difficulties and stroke patients.

additional fluid loss
This may occur in some patients who are taking diuretics as well as in those with fever, diarrhoea, vomiting, burn injury and uncontrolled diabetes. It also occurs immediately following surgery. In winter, central heating can lead to low humidity, increasing the loss of fluid through the skin.

Maintaining a fluid balance chart or recording the fluid input and output can be useful in clinical situations (Figure 2.3.20).

Study activity 6

a. What percentage of body weight is made up of water?
b. Why do elderly people often drink too little?
c. Check how much liquid (from drinks) you take in per day, on average. Does this correspond with your daily requirement?
d. Why is there a risk of dehydration with diarrhoea, vomiting, and excessive use of diuretics and/or laxatives?

8. Vitamins

a. Functions of vitamins
Vitamins are chemical compounds which occur naturally in certain foods and are essential in small quantities for the normal functioning of metabolism in the body. The amounts of vitamins needed to maintain health are normally present in well-balanced diets. Although sailors have known for many years that eating fresh fruit can prevent scurvy, the existence and functions of vitamins have only been known since 1920. In the industrialised world there is generally a sufficient intake of vitamins but the following points are worth noting:
- Vitamin deficiencies can occur during illness and therapy, particularly due to the long-term use of certain medications, chemotherapy or following surgery to the gastrointestinal tract.
- Vitamin deficiencies may possibly play a part in the occurrence of cancer.

– It is possible to take too many vitamins, particularly when vitamin preparations are used. An overdose of vitamins A and D can have negative consequences for our health, and taking too many vitamin C tablets can cause nausea, vomiting, diarrhoea and even the formation of kidney stones in some susceptible people.

Figure 2.3.21
Flora Project for Heart Disease Prevention

The antioxidant vitamins

Vitamins are essential to life. Without a variety of vitamins, our bodies cannot function properly. Lack of certain vitamins can result in poor health.

Now a growing number of scientific studies suggest that a small group of vitamins may play a bigger part than we previously thought in keeping us healthy. Along with other lifestyle changes like quitting smoking and taking more exercise, antioxidant vitamins – often called the 'ACE' vitamins – may help to protect us from coronary heart disease, the leading cause of death in the UK. Evidence also suggests that they may contribute to the prevention of cancer and other diseases. And the best news of all is that we can get them from many of the foods we eat every day.

The 'ACE' vitamins are beta-carotene (which the body converts to vitamin A when needed), vitamin C and vitamin E. They work by neutralising potentially damaging molecules within the body called 'free radicals' which are produced by normal body processes like digestion and breathing. Vitamin E in particular seems to have an important role in protecting against heart disease. Put simply, the more 'ACE' vitamins we eat, the fewer free radicals are left in our bodies to cause damage.

Choosing 'ACE' foods

Foods that are sources of 'ACE' vitamins add colour and enjoyment to any meal and including them in your daily diet needn't increase your shopping bill.

Recent guidelines set out by the EC suggest that our food supply us with at least 60mg of vitamin C (equivalent to one large orange) and at least 10mg of vitamin E every day. ... While there is no separate recommendation for beta-carotene, experts recommend that many individuals increase their intake.

Good Sources of 'ACE' Vitamins

Beta carotene	Vitamin C	Vitamin E
Brightly coloured fruit and vegetables, including:	Citrus fruit	Vegetable oils, especially sunflower oil
Carrots	Blackcurrants	Products made from
Broccoli	Strawberries	sunflower oil, labelled
Tomatoes	Kiwi fruit	'high in polyunsaturates'
Melons	Green leafy vegetables	Whole grain cereals
Yellow and orange	Potatoes	Nuts such as almonds
peppers	Green peppers	and hazelnuts
Peaches		

Typical vitamin E levels in selected vegetable oils

Sunflower	49mg/100g	Rapeseed	22mg/100g
Corn	17mg/100g	Soya	16mg/100g
Peanut	15mg/100g	Olive	5mg/100g

Source: McCance and Widdowson, 5th edition, 1991

'ACE' vitamins in daily meals

With a bit of planning, we can get all the ACE vitamins we need from the foods we eat every day. In addition to eating more of the foods listed in the box opposite, here are some tips to help you get more ACE vitamins:

– Buy little and often if possible. Many of the vitamins contained in fruit and vegetables are lost through long storage.
– Prepare fruit and vegetables just before you eat and try to leave the skin or peel on wherever possible. Prolonged exposure to air can reduce their nutritional value.
– Use oils only once for shallow frying in order to get their maximum nutritional benefit, and be careful not to heat them beyond smoking point. Oils can be re-used for deep frying, but try not to use them more than five times in order to get the best from them.
– There are many different ways of serving vegetables raw or lightly cooked. Try steaming, stir frying or microwaving them, or plunging them into small amounts of boiling water. How about cooked carrot puree with a touch of nutmeg? Or a crunchy grated raw carrot and cabbage salad?

The advantage in getting vitamin E and the other ACE vitamins from your food rather than from a vitamin supplement is that supplements provide only the vitamins listed on the label. You don't get any of the other nutrients naturally present in the food. A carrot, for instance, will provide you with beta-carotene, dietary fibre, some minerals and some energy. Besides, we all need to eat, so it's just a matter of eating a range of the foods we know are good for us.

Vitamin 'E' and heart disease

Coronary heart disease (known as atherosclerosis) results from the build up of fatty deposits in the walls of the arteries leading to the heart, causing them to narrow. These deposits consist mainly of one type of cholesterol.

People with high levels of cholesterol in their blood are usually at greater risk of heart disease. To help reduce the level of cholesterol we should choose a diet that is lower in fat and partially replace foods high in saturates with those high in polyunsaturates.

Recent research has suggested that antioxidant nutrients such as vitamin E may help to destroy harmful free radicals. These substances have been found to trigger damage to the artery wall, especially when high levels of cholesterol are present.

Certain pollutants, such as cigarette smoke and ultraviolet light, create more free radicals in our body, therefore we need to ensure our diet contains a good supply of the antioxidant vitamins, including vitamin E, thereby decreasing our risk of coronary heart disease.

Figure 2.3.22
Vitamins and deficiency diseases

Vitamins	Deficiency diseases	Symptoms	Food source	Risk groups
C (ascorbic acid)	scurvy	bleeding gums, loose teeth, slow healing of wounds	fruit, vegetables	seriously ill people with fever, burns or tumour formation, people who have undergone extensive/ repeated surgery
B1 (thiamin)	beriberi	muscle paralysis, decreased appetite, irritability	brown bread and other wholemeal cereal products, vegetables, pulses, nuts, pork	alcoholics, people who consume a lot of sugar, or products containing sugar, and few wholemeal products
B2 (riboflavin)	ariboflavinosis	skin defects around the mouth and nose, cornea of the eye clouded by blood vessels	milk and other dairy products, bread and other cereal products, meat, green leaf vegetables, eggs, pulses	women who are pregnant or breast-feeding and not consuming a great quantity of dairy products, people with intestinal diseases, alcoholics
B6 (pyridoxine)	anaemia	listlessness, depression, red, flaky skin around nose, mouth and eyes, poor body growth	meat, fish, milk, eggs, brown bread and other cereal products, potatoes, pulses, and particularly bananas	pregnant women, women taking the contraceptive pill (vitamin B6 alleviates some side-effects of 'the pill'), alcoholics
B12* (cobalamin)	pernicious anaemia	neurological defects	meat, liver, fish, eggs, milk and other dairy products	vegans, people who have undergone a total gastrectomy

Vitamins	Deficiency diseases	Symptoms	Food source	Risk groups
folic acid	anaemia	inflamed mucous membrane of digestive tract	meat, liver, kidney, cereal products, vegetables, particularly green leaf vegetables, potatoes, fruit	people with reabsorption disorders, alcoholics, pregnant women, women taking 'the pill'
A	night-blindness and continuing blindness	poor adaptation to darkness, sores on the cornea of the eye (even to the point of destroying the entire eye), stunted growth	milk fat (in milk, cheese, butter), margarine, liver, low fat margarine, fatty fish, carotene (a type of vitamin A) in orange and green vegetables, egg yolk	people who use a lot of laxatives, people with poor fat digestion
D	rickets	deformation of bones and teeth (thickenings at the bone extremities), weak bones	margarine, low fat margarine, liver, egg yolk, fatty fish, milk fat (in full fat milk, cheese, butter)	people who get too little sunlight, dark-skinned children, people with disturbed fat digestion
E	anaemia, muscular degeneration	changes in connective tissue (looks like normal ageing process), instability of membrane structures	oils, fats, eggs, wholemeal bread and other cereal products	people with disturbed fat digestion
K	haemorrhage reduced haemolysis	delayed blood coagulation	green vegetables, liver, oils, potatoes	people who use antibiotics or other medicines which affect the intestinal flora, newborn babies

* The function of vitamin B12 depends on two factors: an intrinsic factor (produced in the stomach) and an extrinsic factor (contained in the vitamin). Only together are they of use to the body. If the intrinsic factor is missing (after a gastrectomy, for instance) anaemia is likely to result.

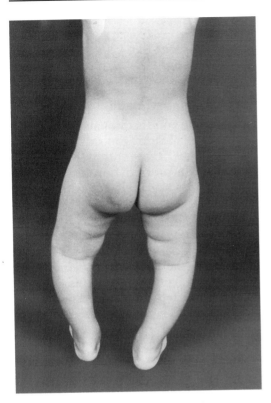

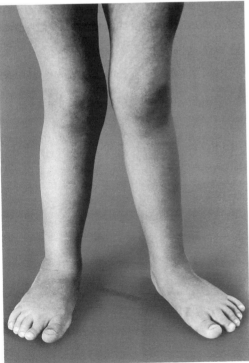

Figure 2.3.23
Vitamin D deficiency may result in decalcification of the skeleton

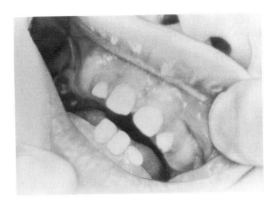

Figure 2.3.24
Bleeding gums can indicate a vitamin C deficiency

Study activity 7

Which statement(s) do you agree with?
All vitamins are equally important.
Long-term deficiency of any vitamin will result in deficiency symptoms.
We should take vitamins during the winter months.
Taking vitamin preparations cannot do any harm and might do some good.
If you are feeling tired and listless, take vitamin preparations.

b. Vitamins in our food
Figure 2.3.22 lists the most significant vitamins, their presence in foodstuffs, and the illnesses and symptoms (known as deficiency diseases) which can occur. It also indicates those groups of the population which are most at risk of suffering from vitamin deficiency.

We can roughly divide the vitamins into two groups:
– the vitamins which are soluble in water: vitamins B1, B2, B6, folic acid and vitamin C.
– the vitamins which are soluble in fat: vitamins A, D, E and K.

9. Minerals

Minerals are naturally occurring solid inorganic substances which are required in the diet to maintain health. They are present in the body in widely varying quantities. A body weight of 60 kilos will contain around one kilogram of calcium and approximately 4 grams of iron. The amount of each separate mineral required in the diet, therefore, also varies greatly.

a. Functions

Minerals are important building substances for the body. For example, calcium makes our bones firm and strong. Minerals, like vitamins, also have a regulatory function in that they help to control the proper function of various processes and systems within the body.

b. Minerals in our food

Important minerals in food are calcium, iron, sodium and iodine. Figure 2.3.25 summarises the most significant ones, and their sources, functions, deficiency symptoms and groups at risk.

> Mrs Simmons is 70 years old and has been a widow for 10 years. Since the death of her husband she has led a very secluded existence. With no children and few friends or acquaintances, she barely has a social life. Recently, she was admitted to hospital with symptoms of dizziness, fatigue and headaches. After various tests it appeared that Mrs Simmons had anaemia based on iron and folic acid deficiency. The registrar consulted the dietitian to take a dietary history in order to trace the deficiencies in the diet. It was found that Mrs Simmons had not eaten a hot meal in the last 10 years because she could not be bothered to cook just for herself. She did not eat cheese, meat or meat products because these were too expensive, and she did not eat brown bread because she preferred white. The dietitian discussed the options for improving her diet, and arrangements were made for her to be able to eat at a local community day centre. Mrs Simmons' situation improved quickly, both physically and socially.

Study activity 8

a. How do you think iron comes to be present in meat?

b. Who will have the greater iron requirement, men or women? Give reasons for your answer.

c. How can your body absorb vitamin D other than through food?

d. Plan a hot meal and a bread-based meal which are rich in iron. Bear in mind that iron is absorbed better into the blood in combination with vitamin C, and that it is not absorbed so well when calcium is present.

e. Which vitamins can be lost into the cooking liquid during preparation? How can you best limit this loss?

f. Make a sketch of the food guide and indicate in what sections the following occur: iron, calcium, vitamin C, thiamin, riboflavin, vitamin B6, folic acid, vitamin B12, vitamin A, vitamin D, vitamin E and vitamin K.

Study activity 9

A 40-year-old woman has been in hospital for two weeks. She gets little physical exercise due to a very complicated leg fracture caused by the accident which resulted in her admission to the hospital. Her typical daily diet consists of the following:

breakfast: 1 slice of brown bread spread with diet margarine and jam, 1 cup of tea with sugar

lunch: 1 portion of soup, 2 potatoes, 1 chicken leg, 2 spoonfuls of gravy (made with cooking fat), 2 spoonfuls of vegetables, a bowl of rice pudding or full fat yoghurt with sugar

tea: 2 slices of brown bread spread with diet margarine, one with cold meat, one with jam, 2 cups of tea with sugar

in between (spread out over the day): 2 cups of coffee with sugar and semi-skimmed milk, 2 biscuits, 1 glass of orange juice (150 ml).

a. Evaluate this diet on the basis of the ten recommendations for a balanced diet.

Figure 2.3.25
Overview of the most important minerals

Mineral	Functions of the body	Deficiency symptoms	Presence in food	Risk groups
calcium	building up the skeleton and teeth, blood coagulation, muscle contraction	bone decalcific-ation (osteoporosis, rickets, weak bones)	particularly in dairy products, green leaf vegetables, cereal products, pulses	elderly people with a vitamin D deficiency, pregnant women
iron	haemoglobin building substance (for oxygen intake and output)	anaemia, muscle fatigue, headache, dizziness	meat, eggs, green vegetables, wholemeal cereal products, pulses	pregnant women, women who are menstruating
sodium	regulation of proper water balance in the body		milk, salt, in all foodstuffs except for sugar and oil, particularly in many ready-made products	people who perspire heavily and for a long time in a warm environment, people suffering from chronic diarrhoea and vomiting
potassium	functioning of the muscles, regulation of a proper water balance in the body	muscle weakness, irregular heartbeat	oranges, bananas, dried fruit, vegetables and almost all other foodstuffs	people who use diuretics and laxatives, people who suffer from severe diarrhoea or vomiting
iodine	building substance of the thyroid gland hormone	slow growth, low metabolism, goitre (enlarged thyroid gland)	drinking water, iodised salt, sea fish, bread, spinach, shellfish	pregnant women, people on a low sodium diet
fluoride	hardening of teeth and bones, protective action against cavities	greater risk of caries	tea, sea fish, drinking water	people who do not use fluoride toothpaste or fluoride tablets

b. For which nutrients does this patient have an increased requirement?

c. How could her diet be improved?

10. Summary

In this chapter we have discussed how food is digested by the body and in what form it reaches the bloodstream. We then looked at the various foods which provide the body's requirements for energy and examined the functions of the most important nutrients together with the consequences of deficiencies or excesses of certain nutrients. We have indicated in which foodstuffs the nutrients can be found and how each food fits into a balanced diet.

Nutrition through the life cycle

1. Introduction

In this chapter, attention will be paid to the special nutritional needs of:
- the infant (up to 1 year old)
- the toddler (1-4 years old)
- the schoolchild (4-12 years old)
- the adolescent (12-20 years old)
- the pregnant woman
- the breastfeeding woman
- the elderly.

The chapter does not discuss normal adult nutrition as this is extensively dealt with in other parts of the book. However, there are different nutritional requirements for optimum health at each stage of life, and these are affected by physical, mental and social factors.

Learning outcomes

After studying this chapter the student should be able to:
- describe the amounts and types of food which can be given to infants;
- explain the deficiencies which can occur in an infant's diet;
- state at least two advantages and two disadvantages each for breastfeeding and bottle feeding;
- suggest three situations where extra fluid must be given to an infant in order to prevent dehydration;
- explain why wheat, oats, barley and rye, may not be added to the infant diet before the sixth month;
- plan a one-day menu for toddlers and explain why it is particularly suitable;
- state three areas which require special attention in the diet of schoolchildren;
- name three factors which can influence an adolescent's diet;
- briefly explain what alcohol does in the body;
- name three nutrients for which pregnant women have an increased requirement and explain the practical implications this has for a pregnant woman's diet;
- explain what polychlorinated biphenyls (PCBs) are, and name three products in which they can be found;

- explain what toxoplasmosis is and how it can be prevented;
- state approximately how much additional energy is required in the diet of a breast-feeding mother;
- give three examples of foodstuffs which can cause stomach cramps in an infant through their presence in mother's milk;
- indicate when it would be better to avoid these foodstuffs;
- state two general causes of poor nutritional status in the elderly;
- describe the attitude of the elderly with regard to nutrition;
- make four recommendations which may help to prevent osteoporosis;
- make several general nutritional recommendations for the elderly and explain why these recommendations are important.

2. Infant nutrition

For the first three months after birth, an infant's nutrition comes only from breast or bottle feeding, or a combination of both. Breastfeeding is generally preferred because of the following factors:

- it is the most 'natural' nutrition, with optimal composition;
- it works to protect against infections and allergies;
- it is always at the correct temperature;
- it encourages psychological and emotional bonding between mother and child.

Bottle feeds may consist of a complete formula milk, sometimes referred to as humanised or modified formula because it resembles mother's milk as closely as possible. Sometimes home-made infant food, such as cow's milk and water mixtures, are used where parents do not wish to use industrially prepared food. Optimal nutrition is important for the substantial growth which an infant undergoes in the first year of life when the child's body weight normally doubles by about 6 months and triples by the end of 12 months.

In cases of fever or diarrhoea, or in especially hot weather, additional fluid intake is important because infants have a large body surface area relative to their weight and can therefore quickly develop dehydration.

After the first three months the infant's diet can be gradually varied, though this is not usually necessary from a nutritional point of view. However, deficiencies in energy, vitamin C, vitamin D and iron can occur after the sixth month if the requirement is greater than can be met by breast or bottle feeding alone. It is also important for the infant to start eating with a spoon to promote jaw development and proper swallowing. The diet can be varied in the fourth month with the addition of fruit and fruit juice, in the fifth month with vegetables and rice, and in the sixth and seventh months with dairy products, fish, meat or meat substitutes, chicken and eggs. Cereals such as barley, oats, and wheat are not recommended before the sixth month because they contain gluten. This protein fraction is implicated in the development of coeliac disease if it is introduced too early.

Initially, foodstuffs are offered as liquid or in a very finely minced/puréed form. Later, when the child develops chewing reflexes (after about 3-4 months) solids can be introduced. For the promotion and maintenance of healthy teeth, it is advisable to give infants as little sugar (either added to or already contained in food) as possible. It may be advisable in some areas to give fluoride supplements to complement the small amount which may be added to drinking water in the UK. In addition, salt should not be added to foods unnecessarily as there may be a risk to young developing kidneys of hypernatraemia.

Figure 2.4.1
Example of a nutritional plan for a healthy infant. The diet can vary, depending on such things as growth, weight, and activity.

During	Number of feeds per day	Begin with
1st month	5-7 bottle-feeds (one of which is usually at night)	breast-feeds, vitamin K shortly after birth by injection, fluoride supplement well spread out over the day; with cow's milk and water mixtures, supplements of vitamins A, D, C and linoleic acid
2nd month	5 breast- or bottle-feeds	" "
3rd month	5 breast- or bottle-feeds	" "
4th month	5 breast- or bottle-feeds, sieved fruit*	vitamin D supplement for breast-fed infants, (diluted) fruit or tomato juice*, mixed fruit*
5th month	4-5 breast- or bottle-feeds, sieved fruit*, hot meal*	easily digestible cooked, mashed vegetables*, jars of baby food, mashed potato, rice, sieved legumes
6th-7th month	2-3 breast- or bottle-feeds after six months, bottle feeds preferably consisting of modified infant feed with extra iron and less protein, porridge**, hot meal	porridge** made with a gluten-free binder such as rice flour (from the sixth month a binder with gluten can be used), 1 spoonful of minced meat, fish, chicken or 1/2 egg, 1 cup of full fat yoghurt (diluted with water at first), crusts of bread from the sixth month, cow's milk
8th month	1 breast- or bottle-feed**, porridge**, 1 bread-based meal with dairy products (milk or full fat yoghurt), 1 hot meal	squares of brown bread with butter and a soft spread
from the 9th month	2 bread-based meals with dairy products (milk or full fat yoghurt), 1 hot meal (possibly 1 breast-feed)	the child learns to drink by itself and is no longer an infant
from the 1st year	milk-feed replaced by full fat milk	

* From a nutritional point of view such supplements are not usually necessary, but they can be used to accustom the child gradually to other food
** Preferably prepared with cow's milk

Study activity 1

   a. Think about the advantages and disadvantages of breastfeeding and bottle feeding for both mother and child, and list them in a table

   b. Which of the following foodstuffs could you give to an infant of six months: fruit juice, custard, mashed banana, spinach, oatmeal porridge, cauliflower, minced beef, crisps, chocolate?

   c. The consumption of milk or full fat yoghurt is recommended for infants. Why?

3. Nutrition for toddlers

There are four main points to consider in toddlers' nutrition. These include the composition of the food, the encouragement of healthy eating habits, the development of the child's taste and awareness of the child's appetite.

a. Composition of the Diet

The proper growth and development of children will be maintained if the composition of the diet is based on the food guide. Figure 2.4.2 suggests the kind of foods that can be used as a basis for healthy eating. Calcium and vitamin D need particular attention because teeth and bones are developing rapidly. To prevent deficiencies and, in particular, rickets, mothers from low income groups may be recommended to give their children vitamin D supplements.

b. Acquiring good eating habits

At this stage of life, the child will acquire basic eating habits. To ensure they are good habits, it is important to teach them to have a proper breakfast, to limit the amount of sweets they eat, to have no more than two or three snacks between meals, and to chew properly. Children should not be allowed to be constantly sucking bottles, cans or cartons filled with soft drinks or fruit juice, as this may lead to dental caries. Parents should also take care not to force food upon children or to use food as a reward or punishment as this can lead to eating disorders and food preferences later in life.

Figure 2.4.2
Daily menu for a toddler

   – brown bread
   – margarine or butter
   – cheese and/or meat product
   – 1 pint (0.5 litres) of milk
   – a small piece of lean meat, fish, chicken, or an egg
   – a generous helping of vegetables
   – potatoes, rice, and pasta as desired
   – at least one helping of fruit
   – carton of yoghurt

c. The development of taste

A child starts to develop its own tastes in food, and parents should take these into account. If, however, the child is allowed too free a choice of food, there is a risk that a very unbalanced diet may result. It is also better for children not to become too accustomed to sweet or salty tastes. Often children may have a good appetite for a narrow range of foods. As the child develops, offer foods previously rejected because these are often accepted on later occasions.

d. Appetite

Because toddlers may have a poor appetite, it is important to provide several small meals over the course of the day. It is also important to ensure that the fat content of the meals is not too high, as fat has a filling effect. Try to make food as interesting as possible and get the child into a routine for meal times.

Study activity 2

   a. Four-year-old Mary has been admitted to the children's ward of a hospital suffering from pneumonia. Her condition has now improved slightly, and she is allowed to eat hot meals. The only vegetables she will eat are baked beans, and her parents say that she refuses to eat any other vegetables at home. How do you deal with this in the hospital?

b. What do you think about toddlers eating sweets and crisps?

c. When parents come to visit their sick children in hospital, what would you recommend that they bring with them as a treat?

d. Discuss some of the reasons why parents give sweets to their children.

Figure 2.4.3
© The Independent 25/11/92

Children's health is threatened by junk food diet

By Liz Hunt
Medical Correspondent

Sweets and soft drinks manufacturers are targeting schools and offering them incentives – such as profit-sharing schemes to raise funds – to stock their products, nutritional experts warned yesterday.

As a result, children have more access to unhealthy food than ever before, threatening their health. In addition, few schools have a policy on what foods are sold on their premises, and many do not monitor nutritional standards of the meals they provide.

A report on children's diets and school meal provision paints a gloomy picture of children growing up on a diet of sweets, fizzy drinks and junk food. It provides the first national guidelines for school meals since the 1980 Education Act removed them. Local education authorities were no longer obliged to provide meals – except for children entitled to free ones – and could determine price and quality themselves.

Crisps, sweets and hot snacks are sold in 90 per cent of schools. Over half of all children buy food at school more than once a week, and one in five buys it every day. Crisps are most common, with a quarter buying two or more packets a day, and nearly half buying two or more chocolate bars or sweets. The growth of fast food outlets has added to the problem. The number of children who eat school dinners is falling – from 64 per cent in 1979 to 42 per cent in 1991 – and many are turning to the high street instead.

Children's diets are high in fat and sugar, low in fibre and some essential vitamins and minerals. Up to 90 per cent of girls are iron deficient, and 93 per cent low in calcium.

Children are suffering from weight problems, dental caries and nutritional anaemia, the report says. But they are also at increased risk of heart disease, cancer and diabetes in later life.

Nutritional Guidelines for School Meals, which has the backing of the Health Education Authority and health organisations, says that many school meals lack nutritional standards. For some children, the school meal is the only hot meal of the day. One in ten children at secondary school has nothing to eat before leaving home, and one in six does not have a hot cooked meal in the evening.

The guidelines, drawn up by the Caroline Walker Trust, which seeks to improve health through good food, set out the energy requirement from 11 key nutrients. It aims to get children eating more bread, cereals and other starchy foods, fruit and vegetables high in vitamins and minerals, and less fat, sugar and salty foods.

School catering has a potential 8.5 million customers each day, said Gill Cawdron, chair of the School Meals Campaign. "If children are to eat healthy school meals, then the challenge will be to provide foods children enjoy."

Nutritional Guidelines for School Meals: P.O. Box 7, London, W3 6XJ; price £8.50.

4. Nutrition for schoolchildren

Schoolchildren, like toddlers, have some specific problems and there are several factors to be noted with regard to their nutritional requirements.

a. Composition of the diet

The composition of the diet should help schoolchildren to achieve optimal growth and development but, because they are generally very active, a relatively large quantity of fuelling substances is needed in addition to an adequate supply of building substances. The ten recommendations for a healthy diet offer useful guidelines in this respect (see Module 2, Chapter 2). Do remember, however, that excessive amounts of dietary fibre may interfere with absorption of some nutrients and should therefore be taken in sensible amounts.

b. School breaks and pocket money

It is recommended that you give children healthy foodstuffs like brown bread, fruit and dairy products to take to school with them for snacks during breaks, or for their midday meal if they cannot come home for lunch. Lots of variety and novelty in the food provided from home can discourage a child from spending pocket money on sweets, crisps or other unsuitable snacks. Parents can also suggest some appealing, non-food alternatives for spending pocket money.

c. Healthy diet and education

Lessons on nutrition in school can encourage children to adopt good eating habits. Figure 2.4.4 shows patterns of eating for Scottish schoolchildren.

Figure 2.4.4
Consumption of foods and non-alcoholic drinks: boys and girls
© RUHBC, The University of Edinburgh, 1992

| | Boys % | | | Girls % | | |
	Daily	Weekly	Rarely	Daily	Weekly	Rarely
Fruit	49.4	35.7	14.9	60.2	31.4	8.4
Raw vegetables	18.3	30.7	51.0	24.8	36.2	39.0
Wholemeal bread	47.8	19.5	32.7	46.9	21.3	31.9
Crisps	61.8	28.4	9.7	66.8	24.9	8.3
Sweets	68.3	25.4	6.3	64.1	28.4	7.5
Chips	35.2	49.6	15.2	26.5	52.4	21.0
Sausages, etc.	19.1	57.3	23.5	10.1	50.4	39.5
Low fat milk	42.6	8.7	48.8	41.6	8.5	50.0
Whole fat milk	58.8	8.6	32.7	48.1	9.0	42.9
Fizzy drinks	69.1	22.5	8.4	62.0	27.1	11.0
Coffee	28.6	15.1	56.3	29.1	12.0	58.9
Tea	53.7	15.9	30.4	52.3	15.1	32.6

The analytic procedure of factor analysis was used to reveal that children's eating is patterned such that frequent eating of chips, crisps, sausages, etc., sweets and sugar-containing fizzy drinks are associated with one another. Frequent eating of fruit, raw vegetables, wholemeal bread and low fat milk are also associated. Thus patterns of 'healthy' and 'unhealthy' eating can be identified in young people.
High fat foods: Crisps are eaten daily by almost $2/3$ of girls and only slightly fewer boys. Chips are eaten every day by over $1/3$ of boys and $1/4$ of girls. One in five boys eats sausages or other high fat content meats daily.
High sugar content foods: Two out of three children consume sweets and sugar-containing fizzy drinks every day.
High fibre foods: Just under half the children eat wholemeal bread daily; around 55% eat fruit daily and under one in 4 eats raw vegetables every day.
Vitamins and minerals: Apart from in fruit, vegetables and wholemeal bread (see above) 84% of children get vitamins and minerals from drinking milk every day (either full fat or semi-skimmed).
Caffeine: Almost $2/3$ of children drink either tea or coffee every day.
Thus, in general, snack foods such as crisps and sweets are a more common part of children's daily diets than is fresh fruit.

Study activity 3

a. Think of some attractive alternatives to sweets for a children's party.

b. Eight-year-old Kevin has been admitted to hospital after a car accident. In order to promote the rapid recovery of his many fractures it is desirable that he eats a lot of dairy products. Kevin is quite happy about this because he drinks a lot of chocolate-flavoured milk and fruit yoghurt, and likes to eat puddings and custard. What is your opinion on these dairy products, and what advice would you give to Kevin?

5. Nutrition for adolescents

Adolescence is a very important stage of life from the point of view of nutrition. During this time the body develops into maturity, and there are, again, specific nutritional considerations which should be addressed.

a. Composition of the diet

Composed with the help of the food guide, the diet should contain the ideal quantities of proteins, vitamins and minerals. Girls generally mature more quickly than boys, and they have less muscle tissue but more fat tissue, which makes their energy requirement lower. Their diet must be balanced in such a way that deficiencies are prevented, and it is particularly important to make sure there is sufficient iron to compensate for the loss of iron during menstruation. Girls often have a greater fear of becoming overweight than boys (indeed, they do gain weight more easily), and this can result in their eating the wrong foods, leading in turn to problems like anaemia, or osteoporosis in later years. In Section 8 of this chapter the causes of and prevention of osteoporosis are discussed. Both boys and girls can be plagued by acne, and while a special diet will not be of much specific help, a healthy, balanced diet is still to be recommended.

b. Group behaviour and alcohol consumption

One of the notable characteristics of this life stage is group behaviour, where adolescents conform to the habits, customs, attitudes, fashions, conduct, and morals of their peers. A great deal has been written about the social, behavioural and psychological aspects of peer pressure. Group behaviour can also exert considerable influence on eating and drinking habits so that adolescents may want to eat and drink the same things as their peers, and this is often how alcoholic drinks are introduced into their diet. Advertising also shows alcohol consumption as being fashionable and sociable. As a result, the incidence of alcohol abuse among adolescents is increasing, and it is vital that they receive sound advice about the proper use of alcohol and the dangers of its misuse.

Figure 2.4.5
A glass of beer contains almost as much pure alcohol as a glass of wine. The glasses are smaller in proportion to the amount of alcohol they contain.

average alcohol percentage in beer	3%
average alcohol percentage in wine	10%
average alcohol percentage in spirits	37%

c. What does alcohol do in our body?

Drinking a few glasses of alcohol a few times a week does not really cause any physical problems. This is because a particular enzyme in our body is capable of making small amounts of alcohol disappear relatively quickly. Drinking too much on occasion can have some negative consequences, for instance, delaying your capacity to react while driving. Long-term alcohol abuse affects the stomach, liver, pancreas, heart and arteries, and can also cause malfunctions in the brain and nervous system. That is why alcoholics often show signs of dementia and lose their short-term memory.

Figure 2.4.6
© The Daily Telegraph 28/6/94

Teenagers must look back to the iron age

*The common adolescent diet may be a nutritional time bomb, finds **Christine Doyle,** affecting academic performance as well as health*

Look closely at any group of palely loitering teenage girls and you might see some borderline candidates for iron deficiency anaemia. They could already suffer marginal symptoms of tiredness, lack of concentration, headaches and exhaustion.

But ask them about healthy eating and you risk a dismissive: "You don't want to get stressed out about that."

The response is familiar to many parents who leave iron supplements on the kitchen table in the hope of redressing an imbalance. Yet increasingly, nutritionists chart worryingly low intakes of iron and low iron stocks in the body, especially in adolescents.

A report last week that cancer rates and heart disease in confirmed vegetarians are much lower than in meat-eaters is encouraging.

However, it should alert us to ensuring that the "veggie generation" eats the right sort of green vegetables and other food to keep up energy. As it is, many drift in and out of a subsistence diet of chips, pizza, crisps and cola.

Iron is vital for the formation of haemoglobin, which carries oxygen around the body: it is also essential for healthy muscles and for some reactions in the brain. Moreover, once adolescent girls menstruate they need extra iron to compensate for the loss in blood.

Yet a recent study, which found that more than one in five 11- to 16-year-olds rarely discussed healthy eating at school, does not inspire confidence. Furthermore, a study of 12- to 14-year-olds in affluent Richmond and Kingston in Surrey disclosed that one in five leaves home without breakfast: more than 16 per cent of girls also skipped lunch.

Detailed scientific studies, such as one carried out among 400 white, middle-class 12- to 14-year-olds at a London school, spell out the problem. Ten per cent of girls and three per cent of boys were anaemic, with haemoglobin counts below accepted normal levels, says Dr Mike Nelson of the nutrition and dietetics department at King's College, London who led the study. Moreover, 15 per cent of boys and girls had borderline iron reserves.

Vegetarians and slimmers are most at risk, with around one in four having signs of anaemia or low iron stocks. They carry three times the risk found in meat-eaters and non-dieters. Iron in red meat and meat products is more readily absorbed than from any other food. Those from deprived backgrounds are also significantly more at risk.

Iron is crucial for normal mental and physical development in the womb and during infancy, and severe deficits can lead to irreversible impairment of mental and physical development.

Teasing out the effects of deficiency on the mental or physical health of teenagers is more complicated, because there are so many environmental and other hormonal influences on their life.

Broader studies link low iron status with reduced immune response to infection, especially in the chronically sick, with poor academic performance and with difficult or disruptive behaviour. Iron supplementation leads to improvements.

Dr Nelson says: "One cannot rule out the possibility that academic and physical performance, as well as health, may be compromised in British school children because of poor iron status."

A new study by Dr Nelson on the physical effects of iron deficiency will focus attention on whether low levels of iron in adolescents, particularly girls, takes the edge off physical stamina and, by extension, off the ability to concentrate at school.

Carried out among 114 11- to 14-year-old girls in a multi-ethnic school in Wembley, it discloses not only that one in five girls is anaemic, but that their heart rates, raised during a step test exercise, recover less efficiently than those of their non-anaemic classmates.

One theory is that some children with low iron stocks may automatically reduce their activity level in order to avoid feeling listless or tired. That could lead them to reduce their academic performance too. It could also lead to future risks, such as less healthy bones, overweight or heart disease. Should the low iron levels persist for several years, as government surveys suggest, there is also the worry that increasing numbers of young women are ill-prepared for pregnancy.

Taking iron supplements during pregnancy may come too late: foetal development is critical during the first few weeks, perhaps before a woman realises she is pregnant.

According to Dr Sue Fairweather-Tait, a principal scientist at the Institute of Food Research in Norwich and a member of a British Nutrition Foundation task force on iron: "There is a strong possibility that iron deficiency is developing into a Nineties' nutritional time bomb."

White and brown bread are already fortified with iron, and one solution, favoured by some scientists, would be an extension to other foods – cynics say that for maximum impact these would have to be crisps, chips or ketchup.

Others argue that fortification is a blunderbuss approach: they point to the decline in children's diets since the abandonment of nutritional standards for school meals in 1980 and call for a return.

A well-balanced school lunch should contain 30 to 40 per cent of the daily iron requirement.

Meanwhile, parents, teachers and teenagers could avert this insidious eating disorder by arming themselves with a few of the ground rules described here.

Extra energy: facts and fallacies

■ **How much iron?** Recommended daily nutrient intake for 1- to 14-year-old boys is 11.3mg and for girls 14.8mg.

■ **The richest sources.** Red meat, liver and kidneys have the highest levels, with poultry and oily fish such as sardines and tuna containing smaller amounts. Green vegetables, bread, cereals, lentils, beans, dried fruit, cocoa and eggs. White bread and cereals are fortified with iron.

■ **The key to understanding iron.** You may, theoretically, have a high intake, but it can go right through you. It depends on the "bioavailability". The iron in lean meat and oil is in a free form chemically, and about 20 per cent is easily absorbed into the body without interference from other chemicals in food.

There is less iron in plants and cereals, and chemically it is in a less free form, which is why vegetarians should plan their meals carefully. Access to the body is also inhibited by other chemicals in food. Spinach, for example, has as much iron as meat, but contains oxalates – the chemicals that cause the "gritty" feel in the mouth. These attract iron and bind it, lowering absorption to as little as 1.4 per cent of the total. Wholegrain cereals contain phytates which also "trap" iron. About five per cent of the iron in pulses and high fibre cereals to which iron has been added is absorbed. Processed bran, such as All-Bran, contains fewer phytates than the unprocessed variety that you sprinkle on food.

■ **Why Vitamin C is crucial.** Drink fresh orange or vitamin C-enriched soft drink with a meal and it will "unlock" captive iron. The vitamin attracts iron to it but less lightly than phytates or oxalates, making absorption easier.

Nutritionists say the importance of vitamin C for boosting iron bio-availability cannot be stressed enough. In the study of middle-class children 14.5 per cent were anaemic where both iron and vitamin C intakes were low compared with 2.3 per cent where iron and vitamin C intakes were high.

■ **The Importance of a good breakfast.** Adolescents who eat cereals four or more times a week take nearly a third more iron than those who eat cereals fewer than three times a week. Consumption of crisps, chips and fizzy drinks reduces hunger for balanced iron-rich meals and leads to iron deficiency.

■ **What about tea or coffee?** The tannins inhibit iron absorption. Take tea with your breakfast cereal and two per cent of the iron is absorbed. Substitute fruit juice and around eight per cent will get through. Fizzy drinks, similarly, contain phosphates which may reduce iron absorption.

■ **Is Guinness good for you?** Despite its bodybuilding reputation, Guinness contains virtually no iron, according to Sue Fairweather-Tait of the Institute for Food Research in Norwich. But both red and white wine contain iron with absorption from white wine said to be up to 10 per cent. Apparently alcohol increases the intestine's permeability to iron and may contain substances which, like vitamin C, stimulate iron absorption.

■ **Was Popeye right?** Even though spinach contains a lot of iron, Popeye's reputation was at least helped by the slip of a decimal point by a food analyst which led to a tenfold increase in the estimated amount of iron in spinach.

■ **Should you take a supplement?** Depleted iron reserves are so prevalent among adolescent vegetarians, especially in a meat-eating household, that supplements are advisable. Likewise dieting adolescents could be well advised to take an iron pill. Official figures show that 16 per cent of women and three per cent of men have negligible iron reserves. But Dr Fairweather-Tait says exercise is preferable to taking supplements: "Then you will feel hungry, eat more and take in more iron."

■ **Computer risk.** Youngsters who sit for hours at computers may eat less, putting themselves at risk of deficiency.

■ **Does anaemia show in the "pinks" of your eyes?** An old test but not valid unless there is a change over a period of time from pink to a drained white. Better to ask your doctor for a blood test if you are feeling run-down, lacking in energy and more tired than usual.

Iron Rations

These two menus, one with meat and one vegetarian, allow for more than the required daily intake of iron for 15-year-olds. The menus are also in line with a daily energy requirement officially estimated at 2,110kcal.

Lean Meat Menu

Breakfast: two Weetabix; 1/2 pt of semi-skimmed milk; two slices of wholemeal toast with a scraping of margarine; one glass of fresh orange.

Mid morning: one apple.

Lunch: two wholemeal sandwiches (four slices/rounds bread) with a scraping of margarine and a filling of lean ham and salad; a low calorie yoghurt and a small banana.

Mid afternoon: two plain digestive biscuits.

Evening meal: medium portion of spaghetti bolognaise with wholemeal spaghetti (220g); boiled or steamed carrots and green beans; baked apple with sultanas.

Late evening: four wholemeal crackers; Edam cheese (60g).

Vegetarian Menu

Breakfast: two Weetabix; 1/2 pt of semi-skimmed milk; two slices of wholemeal toast with a scraping of margarine; one glass of fresh orange.

Mid morning: one apple or dried apricots.

Lunch: baked beans (135g) on toast (four rounds) with a scraping of margarine and a grilled tomato; a low calorie yoghurt and a small banana.

Mid afternoon: two plain digestive biscuits.

Evening meal: 100g grilled nut cutlet, boiled or steamed carrots and green beans; baked apple with sultanas.

Late evening: four wholemeal crackers; Edam cheese (60g).

Menus supplied by the Meat and Livestock Commission's senior nutritionist.

---

d. Appetite and the consumption of sweets and snacks

Adolescents often have big appetites. In order to satisfy their hunger between meals they often consume snacks rich in fat, sweets rich in energy, drinks with a high sugar content, or alcohol. More significantly, intakes vary greatly from day to day. Cafeterias in schools, workplaces and sports facilities can contribute to the improvement of adolescents' eating behaviour by offering healthy snacks and drinks for sale.

e. Critical view of society

Adolescents' diets may also be affected by their view of society. For instance, they might refuse to eat meat for moral reasons, or they may become concerned about the effects of the additives such as preservatives, colouring agents, hormones and aroma and flavour enhancers which are found in many foods. This can result in some adolescents adhering to an alternative diet (see Module 4, Chapter 1). The search for their own identity may also result in a change in eating habits.

Study activity 4

a. Name some healthy and tasty foodstuffs which can serve as substitutes for snacks, sweets, soft drinks and alcoholic beverages in a sports club cafeteria.

b. Ann is 15 years old and studying for her exams. She is overweight and would very much like to lose weight. For lunch she eats:
   - 2 slices of white bread, with margarine, corned beef and tomato ketchup
   - a packet of crisps
   - a bar of chocolate
   - 1 cup of tea with milk and 2 spoons of sugar

   Make some suggestions as to how she could change her lunch diet in order to lose some weight. Explain the changes that you have recommended.

6. Nutrition for pregnant women

The following points are important for ensuring optimal nutritional status in both the pregnant woman and the foetus.

Figure 2.4.7
Baby Building Foods. © Manitoba Health

Baby building foods

Nature has given you nine months to lay a solid foundation for your child. What you eat while you are pregnant will affect your baby for the rest of its life.

Remember these nutrition tips:
– have four milk servings daily
– have five bread and cereal servings daily
– have two meat and alternate servings daily
– have five fruit and vegetable servings daily
– eat frequent snacks, particularly before bedtime
– gain 11-13kg (24-29lb)

To feed your baby after birth, breastfeeding is best. It allows you to continue to build on the solid foundation you started during pregnancy.

a. Composition of the diet

A properly formulated diet is necessary for the growth and development of the foetus and for the maintenance of the mother's body. No special nutritional requirements exist during the first six months of pregnancy, but that does not mean that good dietary status during this time is not important. After the first six months, there is an increased need for protein, calcium, iron, vitamins and energy. In addition to the recommendations of the food guide and the ten recommendations for a balanced diet, the additional daily consumption of 1 glass of milk or 1 slice of cheese, 1 slice of bread or 1 potato and 1 portion of fruit is desirable.

By limiting fat and sugar in the diet (and definitely not 'eating for two'), obesity can be prevented. Obesity during pregnancy increases the risk of complications like gestational hypertension and diabetes, and the weight should not increase by more than 20% of the 'ideal' body weight during pregnancy. Restricting fatty meat, fatty fish and full fat dairy products is also recommended during pregnancy (and at other times) because of the presence of PCBs (polychlorinated biphenyl) in these foodstuffs. These are toxic chemicals which occur in lubricants, glue, and softening agents for resins, lacquers and plastics. These fat-soluble toxic substances collect in the liver and in the fat tissue of humans and animals and they can cause skin defects, pimples, strong pigmentation, jaundice, liver damage, neurological defects and cancer.

b. Hormonal changes

Hormonal changes during pregnancy can lead to nausea and vomiting, particularly during the first three months, and frequent small meals and a light breakfast (such as toast) can help. The hormonal changes can also affect the function of the colon, causing constipation, so food high in dietary fibre and a sufficient fluid intake are essential.

c. Changes in taste

Some pregnant women develop peculiar likes and dislikes in foodstuffs, such as a preference for acidic foodstuffs like pickles or an aversion to coffee.

d. Alcohol consumption

There is no scientific evidence to support the view that one or two alcoholic drinks a day will not do any harm during pregnancy. It is best to avoid alcohol altogether, particularly in the first three months of the pregnancy when the infant's organs are being formed. Excessive alcohol consumption during pregnancy can lead to mental retardation and the child being underweight.

e. Moderate use of salt and very salty foodstuffs

During pregnancy the body is more likely to retain water and the woman is more likely to suffer from hypertension, which in turn can lead to toxaemia. In order to prevent this, it is recommended that salt and very salty foodstuffs are consumed only in moderation.

f. Avoiding raw and medium-rare meat

Toxoplasmosis is an illness which causes serious permanent damage to the organs of the foetus (in particular, brain and eye defects) through a micro-organism that occurs in raw and medium-rare meat.

g. Avoiding soft cheeses

Listeriosis occurs sporadically in the UK. The disease is usually food-borne and is caused by the micro-organism Listeria monocytogenes which contaminates particularly soft cheeses such as Camembert and Brie. It may cause septicaemia or meningitis in either the pregnant mother or the foetus, or lead to early abortion or stillbirth. Soft cheeses such as those mentioned are therefore best avoided.

Figure 2.4.8
© The Times 6/6/92

Study activity 5

a. Considering the recommendation about salty foods, what advice would you give to a pregnant woman who finds it very difficult to eat unsalted food?

b. Plan a one-day menu for a woman who is seven months pregnant.

c. Think of two reasons why a woman should not try to lose weight during pregnancy, even if she is overweight.

You are what they ate

For 20 years, nutritionists have been insisting that healthy eating is the key to avoiding heart disease. But, Nigel Hawkes argues, recent findings suggest that our chances of survival are more likely to depend on the diet of our mothers.

Why are the French so healthy? Nouvelle cuisine notwithstanding, they enjoy a diet which is at least as rich in animal fats as anything eaten in Britain or the United States. The nation that gave the world Béarnaise sauce and glories in the production of more than 250 cheeses cannot be accused of dietary wimpishness: yet heart disease kills only half as many Frenchmen as it does Britons or Americans. It hardly seems fair.

Le Paradoxe français, as it is known to students of heart disease, is now the subject of careful scrutiny. For some reason which many people would love to understand, the French have become the national equivalent of those annoying individuals who break all the dietary rules and get away with it. A Gascon diet rich in fat and flavour does not have the same terrible consequences as a Scottish, Finnish, English, Irish, Australian or American diet.

The Gascons, indeed, exemplify the French paradox. They live in an area famed for the production of pâté de foie gras; and if food were judged by a board of censors, that would qualify as hard-core. According to Serge Renaud, director of research at the Institut National de la Santé et de la Recherche Médicale in Lyons, they eat a diet higher in animal fats than any other group in the developed world. Yet World Health Organisation figures show that Gascons have the lowest rate of heart disease in France. The disease carries off only 80 middle-aged men per 100,000 in Toulouse, against almost 400 in Glasgow.

Figures such as these make one pause. Twenty years of teaching by doctors, healthy-eating proponents and government departments have convinced most of us that our diets are deadly. The central villain has been identified as animal fat, the source of the cholesterol that leads to clogging of the arteries. The propaganda has been effective: opinion polls show that in 1982 only 6 per cent of those questioned in Britain mentioned high cholesterol levels as a cause of heart attacks, but by 1989 the number had risen to 70 per cent. Seldom has any medical theory become accepted wisdom with such impressive speed.

The odd thing is that this has happened without the solid consensus of medical opinion which it presupposes. There have always been individuals willing to point out that the facts do not all support the hypothesis, but they have been brushed aside. Dietary correctness rules.

Habits, however, have changed more slowly than attitudes. The amount of energy in the diet provided by fat has fallen hardly at all in the past 20 years, yet over the same period heart disease *has* fallen in all developed countries, including Britain. The picture is one of death rates rising steeply in the Fifties and Sixties, peaking in the late Sixties, then beginning to fall equally fast. Against that, the curve of fat consumption has been virtually flat, with no hint of the dramatic rise and fall one would expect if there really was the close link we have been led to expect.

The temptation is to throw the dietary hypothesis out of the window, uttering shrill cries. This was, roughly, the import of a recent book published by the Social Affairs Unit (*Health, Lifestyle and Environment: Countering the Panic*), which pointed out, inter alia, that the promoters of a healthy diet have a notoriously inconsistent aim.

In the Thirties, John Boyd Orr – later Lord Boyd Orr, and a Nobel prize-winner – promoted the idea of milk, meat and dairy products as a healthy diet, pointing out that wealthy children grew taller than poor ones. In 1938, the British Medical Association recommended that people should drink 80 per cent more milk, and eat 30 per cent more meat, 55 per cent more eggs and 40 per cent more butter.

Today, of course, the BMA is singing a very different tune; or, rather, the same tune but different words. The message that we are to blame for the things that happen to us is unchanged, but today's evangelists say we are eating too much fat, while yesterday's lamented that we ate so little.

A survey carried out by Mori for the National Dairy Council showed that the public is confused by the conflicting messages. Unsurprisingly, the council concluded that the "eat less fat" message had been overemphasised, and produced advice of its own that amounted to the adage, "A little of what you fancy does you good". By this time, alas, many people may have stopped listening.

The urge to ignore all advice should, however, be resisted; for there is now interesting evidence that may explain some of the paradoxes that heart disease keeps throwing at us. But first, what evidence is there that fat is responsible for heart disease, and will we really prolong our lives by following the currently fashionable advice?

The Committee on the Medical Aspects of Food Policy (COMA) claimed in the Eighties that comparisons between countries show "a strong positive relationship between the proportion of dietary energy derived from saturated fatty acids and mortality from heart disease". As the French figures show, this is very far from obvious. Nor is it clear even within Britain that the regional variations in heart disease can be correlated with fat consumption. The figures can even be used to show that the opposite is true, with the highest consumption of fats in the Southeast and East Anglia, where heart disease deaths are lowest, and the lowest in Scotland, where they are highest. For a "disease of affluence", as heart disease is so often described, it shows a remarkable tendency to crop up most often in the least affluent parts of the country. How can a belief that flies so directly in the face of the facts have established itself so securely?

The origin of the fat hypothesis derives from the work of the American Ancel Keys, who, in a series of studies in the Sixties, appeared to show that the Mediterranean diet – relatively small quantities of meat eaten with volumes of pasta – produced a much lower number of heart deaths than the north European diet. While it is true that fewer people die of heart disease in Italy than in Britain, such comparisons cannot in themselves demonstrate that fat is the cause.

Lung cancer death rates show exactly the same variations, even though levels of smoking are much the same across Europe. The Greeks, for example, smoke just as much as the British, but suffer much less lung cancer. Even more strikingly, the Japanese, whose cigarette consumption considerably exceeds that in any European country, show only a fraction as much lung cancer. The truth is that different countries apparently have different susceptibilities to different diseases, for reasons that are not understood.

Nobody, of course, has ever claimed that fat is the sole cause of heart disease. Conventionally, doctors talk in terms of "risk factors", of which the cholesterol produced by eating a diet high in saturated fats is only one. The others include heredity, obesity, high blood pressure, and lack of exercise while also reducing cholesterol acts on several of these risk factors at once, so does not depend entirely on the alleged link between fats and heart disease. We might thus hope that such changes would make a dramatic difference; but once again, the evidence is far from clear-cut.

Moderate changes in diet seldom have very significant effects on cholesterol levels. Professor Lawrence Ramsay of the Hallamshire Hospital in Sheffield reviewed the results of such diets and found that even cutting total fat by roughly a quarter reduced blood cholesterol by only a couple of percentage points. Better results were obtained with more rigorous diets, with reductions in the range from 6 to 15 per cent.

When the effect of such regimes on death rates is studied, however, a curious result emerges. While diets and cholesterol-reducing drugs do reduce the number of heart attacks and deaths from heart disease, they do not reduce overall death rates. Professor Matthew Muldoon of the University of Pittsburgh reviewed the results of six such trials, covering 120,000 person-years of observation and treatment, and could find no decrease in overall mortality. What was gained in reduced heart mortality was lost in an increase in deaths through suicide, accident or violence.

Other investigators had found the same effect but dismissed it as pure chance. When all the studies were added together by Muldoon, however, he showed that the increase in these categories of death was indeed significant. In the American population as a whole, murders, suicides and car accidents claim 62 men out of every 100,000 in the 45 to 54 age group. Among those on cholesterol-lowering diets or drugs, the number was 107, sufficient to wipe out the relatively modest reductions in heart deaths. In the treated groups, 28 fewer died of heart disease and 29 more from suicide, murder or accident. So, if the reduction in heart deaths is to be taken as a significant result, as the cholesterol campaigners urge, so must the increase in violent deaths.

Nobody has yet come up with a complete explanation of this finding. One possibility, suggested in a recent issue of *The Lancet* by Dr Hyman Engelberg of Cedars-Sinai Medical Center, in Los Angeles, is that lowering cholesterol may increase the amount of a brain chemical, serotinin, whose function in the nervous system is to control aggressive behaviour. If he is right, then reducing cholesterol could seriously damage your mental stability.

Be that as it may, a careful look at the evidence fails to convince me that the dietary hypothesis, as conventionally put forward, can be right. One who agrees is Professor David Barker, of the Medical Research Council's environmental epidemiology unit at Southampton University. "Every day we get fresh evidence that the cholesterol hypothesis doesn't explain heart disease," he says. Fortunately, Barker has come up with a new theory which resolves many of the paradoxes, and could revolutionise our view, not only of heart disease, but of other degenerative diseases as well.

Barker and his colleagues believe the key lies in the womb and in the first year of life.It is then, they say, that a pattern is established which will determine the individual's chances of suffering a heart attack 50, 60 or 70 years later. The theory begins from the observation that the places which now have high mortality from heart disease and strokes are the same as those that, a generation or two ago, had high infant mortality rates.

So is it perhaps some feature of the earliest stages of life that determines our chances of heart disease? Barker has been fortunate to find caches of evidence, in old obstetric records, that enable him to compare such things as weight at birth and weight at any one year with subsequent medical history. In Hertfordshire, the records were begun in 1911 by a far-sighted chief health visitor who insisted that every baby born in the country should be weighed. Later, similar records were begun in a hospital in Preston.

The Hertfordshire records quickly demonstrated an extraordinary fact. By tracing the subsequent life history of 6,500 men, Barker was able to find that their weight at one year of age was a more accurate way of predicting their death from heart disease than cholesterol measurements done within a year or two of their deaths. The lighter babies showed a much higher risk than the heavier ones.

Looking at the Preston figures, where the weight of the placenta was recorded as well as that of the baby, he found that babies who were relatively small in relation to the placenta were more likely to suffer from high blood pressure. The evidence is that dietary influences in the womb and in the first year of life can establish a pattern which influences the kind of disease that may be suffered decades later.

Barker and his team have created a new model for the dietary causes of heart disease. An infant adapted in the womb and the first year of life to a poor diet is, on this view, more vulnerable to affluence when he or she later meets it. This theory helps to explain many puzzles that are otherwise inexplicable.

For example, it explains why death rates from heart disease are now falling, but on a timetable that is different in different countries. Barker suggests that the improvement in diet among expectant mothers happened sooner in the US than it did in the UK, and sooner in more prosperous areas of Britain than in poorer ones. As a result, the poorer areas have been slower to feel the benefits of better maternal nutrition.

The theory might also explain the wide disparities between different countries, even the French paradox. If we assume that Gascon peasants have always eaten well, then, according to Barker's thesis, their babies will be well-adapted to a rich diet. They will not suffer the same consequences from eating it as would a child born elsewhere, to a differently nourished mother.

He suggests that there are critical moments in the development of the foetus and the infant when the organs are being formed, windows of opportunity which, once missed, cannot be recaptured. A foetus starved of nutrients will tend to concentrate efforts on ensuring that the brain, the most vital organ of all, is protected, at the cost of other organs; sure enough, babies whose heads are large in proportion to the rest of their bodies in Barker's archive do badly in the heart disease stakes later in life.

The thesis has not been without its critics, who say that the Southampton team has failed to pay sufficient attention to continuing disadvantage among low birth-weight babies. The critics' argument is that low birth-weight and low weight at one year are indicators of general social disadvantage, which is reflected in many diseases, not simply heart disease. Against that, however, must be set the fact that the Barker findings are very specific. The variations he has found do not appear to act on all the risk factors at once: some appear to contribute to high blood pressure, some to high cholesterol levels, some to sugar intolerance and, eventually, diabetes. And when Barker looks at the link between early weight and heart disease risk factors, he finds them to be independent of social class.

The possibility is, as Roger Robinson, an editor of the *British Medical Journal*, wrote in a recent editorial, that we may be witnessing what the historian of science Thomas Kuhn called "a paradigm shift", when an old theory is replaced wholesale by a new one better able to explain the facts. Such events happen rarely in science, but the confusion over heart disease is so complete that the subject is ready for a revolution.

If Barker is right, what should individuals do about it? It may seem that our fate is fixed by what our mothers ate before we were born, and what they gave us to eat in our first year of life, and there is nothing we can do about it; but that is not quite the right conclusion to draw.

The correct response would seem to be more complex. It is that if we belong to the groups disadvantaged by their early experiences, then a "healthy eating" diet may well be our best option,

for our systems are not programmed to take anything richer. If, on the other hand, our mothers were as well-fed as the Gascons, then we have no special reason to deny ourselves the same kind of food. The trouble is, of course, that we do not really know how well our mothers ate, or even what "eating well" means in this context.

Of one thing we probably can be sure. Diets for expectant mothers did improve in Britain in the Forties and Fifties, first in the war and later as a result of the welfare state, so the cohort of children born in that era should show much lower levels of heart disease. The fall in deaths may be hastened, though not by very much, by the adoption of healthier diets. What really does matter, if Barker is right, is that plenty of effort be devoted to devising the best possible diets for pregnant women and for their babies; for here it seems, may lie the key not only to heart disease but to many other conditions as well.

© Times Newspapers Ltd 1992

Figure 2.4.9
Your First Baby, © The Royal College of Midwives. 1992. London

Feeding your baby

Breastfeeding

Breastfeeding is the most natural way to feed a baby and most mothers find it very enjoyable. Do think seriously about it.

■ **Nourishment.** Breast milk has the right substances – protein, fats, carbohydrates and minerals for your baby. It is made with the type of ingredients which can be easily digested and easily used by the baby's body. It has the right balance of fluid and varies in strength at different times of day to suit the baby's needs.

■ **Growth.** Breast milk contains exactly the right proteins to build the baby's body, so that the growth which takes place is of firm muscles and flesh. The fat in breast milk is used more for energy and warmth and less for growth. This means the breastfed baby does not become flabby and fat.

■ **Health.** Breast milk is clean. It is very difficult for it to become infected, which means no upset stomach from feeding. When she breastfeeds her baby, a mother passes on immunity to infections which she has had. Colostrum (early milk) is particularly rich in the antibodies which protect against infection.

Very important – breast milk contains other antibodies which build up the baby and help to stop him from developing allergies such as asthma and eczema. If you breastfeed because there is a family history of asthma or eczema, you should continue to do so for at least six months. If you plan to return to work early, express your milk so that it can be given to the baby by bottle.

■ **Enjoyment ■ Love ■ Security.** These come naturally – the milk is at body temperature, and you and your baby will come close together at each feed. He will get used to your touch and smell and you will become very familiar with the touch of his hands and face against your body. What better way of enjoyable feeding? And what better way for the baby to learn about love and security?

■ **Bonuses.** And breastfeeding has some bonuses! The extra fat which your body carries in pregnancy is used up when milk is made. The sucking of the baby makes the womb contract. This helps it to go back to its normal size more quickly and helps to stop any infection developing. And lastly – **breastfeeding is free!**

7. Nutrition for breastfeeding women

The optimum diet for women who are breastfeeding has many similarities with the diet for pregnant women. Some aspects of it are discussed below.

a. Composition of the diet

Increased dietary requirements must be taken into account at this time, both for the recovery of the mother and for the provision of the infant's food. Extra energy, protein, vitamins and minerals are needed to produce around 900 ml of breast milk per day, which provides approximately 3,360 kJ (800 kcal). As during pregnancy, the consumption of fatty meat, fatty fish, and full fat dairy products is discouraged in view of the PCBs which can be absorbed into the mother's milk. The PCB content of mother's milk is actually higher than that of cow's milk, but fortunately it is not too high. The consumption of sufficient vegetable fat is necessary for the provision of vitamin D.

b. Fluid intake

A woman who is breastfeeding has an increased fluid requirement, and should drink at least 2 to 2.5 litres per day.

c. The consumption of hot spices and foodstuffs with flatulence-inducing and laxative effects

Certain substances from these foods can be absorbed in the mother's milk and can cause cramps in the infant. If the child does suffer from cramps, it is best to cut out spicy foods, and cut down on pulses and legumes which may be the cause of the problem. This reaction can differ substantially between individual children.

d. The consumption of foodstuffs which stimulate the production of mother's milk

Aniseed, dill, fennel and brown ale or stout are said to stimulate the production of mother's milk. However, there is no scientific evidence to support this premise.

Study activity 6

Compile a one-day diet for a breastfeeding mother.

8. Nutrition for the elderly

The living and eating habits of the elderly vary enormously. Many older people are fit, have active social lives, and eat well. However, there are also many who are lonely, or who have suffered mental or physical deterioration (or both), and these factors can affect both eating habits and the processing of foods in the body.

Figure 2.4.10
"Age Concern" published in Good Food (March, 1994) (edited) © Good Food 1994

> The majority of older people are not undernourished, so they can afford to eat enough food and are in reasonable health. However, up to one tenth of elderly persons could be at risk – those who are ill, frail or convalescing. Recent research (a study of free living people in sheltered housing in Edinburgh) in 1994 showed that individuals living alone tend to be malnourished. Further, it has been found that three-quarters of those studied suffered from at least mild malnutrition. None of these studies, for example, exceeded the lowest recommendations for acceptable nutrient intake for most nutrients. Most were deficient in vitamins B_6 and vitamin D. Energy intakes were also found to be surprisingly low.

The researchers in Figure 2.4.10 believe that exercise is important in maintaining body weight and stimulating appetite. This will enhance consumption of a wider range and greater amount of micronutrients.

Much of this research is substantiated by a previous government publication (Committee on Medical Aspects of Food Policy – COMA) published in 1992, where the diet of the elderly in care is described as "often inadequate". The report recommends that most people over the age of 65 years should adopt the healthy eating guidance advised for younger adults: eat more dietary fibre (fruit, vegetables and cereal), eat less fat and salt.

a. Dietary status among the elderly
Poor nutritional status among the elderly is not unusual. Reasons may include physical factors (such as problems with chewing), but a decreasing independence and, therefore, a decreasing ability to provide for their own nutritional requirements may also play a role. Poor eyesight or arthritis may be partly responsible, but the ability to cater for personal nutrition may suffer because of loneliness, which can result in a lack of interest in eating. Mental deterioration can result in a person simply forgetting to eat. The reduced nutritional status which may result from all this will lead to an acceleration of the ageing process, during which time fewer new cells are formed while old cells die more quickly.

On the other hand, sometimes food becomes more important as one gets older, and there may be a tendency to eat more than the body needs. Food may assume a greater role in keeping elderly people busy or helping to organise their day and this may result in overeating.

b. Knowledge of and attitude about nutrition
Elderly people may not know very much about healthy eating because they grew up at a time when much less was known about proper nutrition. When they were younger, for example, foods such as butter and bacon and other dairy and meat products, which we now believe should only be eaten in moderation, were in fact widely regarded as good and healthy eating. The elderly may also be unfamiliar with much of the food available today, and this may lead to a lack of variety in the diet and many of them will be more used to worrying about whether they have enough to eat than about variety and balance. Many elderly people are also set in their eating habits being accustomed to using lots of fat and sugar in their foods and tending to overcook things.

Sometimes a special diet is followed for medical reasons. These may include diabetes mellitus, hypertension, and constipation, and although such a diet need not form any obstacle to tasty and varied meals, problems can occur. These diets often require intensive supervision by the doctor, dietitian, or medical staff. Obviously, there is no point in the diet unless it actually contributes to the well-being of the elderly person and he is actually motivated to follow it.

c. Physical changes and nutritional advice
As a person ages, a number of changes occur in the body which influence the nutritional requirements:
- The need for energy decreases because, as one gets older, the metabolism slows down and the elderly tend to take part in less physical activity. However, the need for proteins, minerals and vitamins remains the same. In practice, this means that a person should take less sugar, fewer sweet products, and fewer products rich in fat;
- The adaptive capacity of the digestive tract decreases and chewing problems can occur due to the deterioration of the teeth or to poorly fitting dentures. The elderly often avoid meat, wholemeal bread, fruit and raw vegetables, resulting in vitamin or mineral deficiencies or constipation. Food that is difficult to digest is not tolerated as well, causing difficulties in the gastro-intestinal tract and resulting in problems such as diarrhoea and flatulence. Food poisoning, which would only cause stomach pain and diarrhoea in a young adult, could actually be fatal for an elderly person;
- There is a greater loss of fluid through the skin because the skin has become thinner. This occurs particularly during the winter months in houses with central heating. In addition, elderly people are less thirsty and sometimes drink less for fear of incontinence. Health care workers should pay extra attention to the total daily fluid intake of elderly people, and recognise any signs of dehydration such as lack of appetite, drowsiness, and confusion;

– The elderly often suffer from constipation. This can be caused by decreased physical activity, a fluid intake which is too low, too little dietary fibre, medication which causes constipation, or defects in the large intestine. Extra attention should therefore be paid to the presence of sufficient dietary fibre and fluid in the diet of an elderly person. In practice, this means a diet with plenty of wholemeal bread, vegetables, pulses, legumes, and fruit;

– Elderly people have a greater risk of bone fractures due to osteoporosis, which is a process of bone decalcification occurring particularly amongst people over the age of 60. It is estimated that 25% of women and 10% of men over 65 suffer from osteoporosis, and in order to slow down its progress, it is important that people obtain sufficient calcium (particularly in milk and other dairy products) and vitamin D (particularly from sunlight and in butter, margarine, low fat margarine, egg yolk, and fatty fish). Vitamin D deficiencies are common amongst the elderly, particularly among those living in old people's and nursing homes, and the most significant cause is insufficient exposure to sunlight. If it is impossible for residents to go outdoors, then extra attention must be paid to the amount of vitamin D in the diet and, if necessary, a vitamin D supplement will have to be provided.

Whilst diet can do little to correct osteoporosis, it can certainly help to prevent the disease. The following recommendations are important in this respect:

– sufficient dairy products should be consumed to provide enough calcium (around 2 glasses of milk or yoghurt and 1-2 slices of cheese a day);

– avoid excessive use of animal protein, particularly meat;

– go outdoors regularly. Exposure of the face and arms to sunlight for an hour a week in itself provides sufficient vitamin D. Butter, margarine, low fat margarine, fatty fish, and egg yolk also contain vitamin D;

– if possible, engage in a reasonable amount of physical activity as this slows down bone decalcification;

– cut down on smoking (or better still, stop altogether). Smoking has a negative effect on bone density.

The younger a person is when taking heed of these recommendations, the lesser the chance of osteoporosis occurring in later life. Even for those already suffering from osteoporosis, it is advisable to follow these recommendations in order to slow down the process of bone decalcification as much as possible.

Study activity 7

Do the elderly have a different need for nutrients compared with young adults? Give an explanation for your answer.

Figure 2.4.11
Summary of the nutritional recommendations for the elderly

Nutritional recommendations for the elderly:

– increase consumption of foodstuffs rich in dietary fibre, such as wholemeal bread, pulses, legumes, vegetables and fruit

– drink 2 glasses of milk or yoghurt and eat approximately 1-2 slices of cheese a day

– drink at least 1 litre of liquid a day

– eat a portion of meat or fish, or a suitable substitute, one per day

– reduce consumption of butter, margarine, mayonnaise and other foodstuffs rich in fat, such as cake, biscuits, and fatty meat

– limit consumption of sugar and sweet foods.

d. Appetite
If there is little appetite, a cup of tea or an aperitif a half-hour before a meal may help to stimulate the secretion of gastric juices.

An attractively presented meal and a nicely laid table in a pleasant environment can also be a great help in stimulating the appetite.

e. Meals

Special arrangements can be made for elderly people living on their own who are unable to make their own hot meals. Voluntary organisations such as Meals on Wheels can deliver hot, inexpensive meals to their homes. These meals, often prepared in the kitchens of nursing homes or hospitals, can sometimes be collected by the elderly people themselves, or by their friends. Sometimes the elderly in the neighbourhood can make use of the dining facilities in local day centres. This type of arrangement has the great advantage that it allows the elderly to live on their own for as long as possible and the daily visit to the day centre gives them the opportunity of getting out of the house and meeting people in a similar situation to themselves.

Study activity 8

a. An 80-year-old woman likes her dinner of stew, gravy, carrots and mashed potato all mixed up together. Can you explain why this might be? Do you find this a reasonable eating habit?

b. A 78-year-old man says to you, "For me, food without salt just isn't food. Last year I had to follow a diet which limited sodium and fat intake, but I still eat the same amount of salt on my food and eat chocolate and cakes just as before. So I kick the bucket a little bit sooner, so what?" How would you react to this? Do any of your acquaintances have this same attitude to eating habits?

9. Summary

At every stage of life there are specific nutritional factors which need to be addressed. The nutritional requirements of infants and toddlers are primarily aimed at growth and development. For women who are pregnant or breastfeeding, there are additional nutritional requirements to maintain the mother's health and to promote the growth of the foetus or infant. Growth and development of the body demand a great quantity of building substances. For the elderly, the building substances are needed for the maintenance or acquisition of good nutritional status. The goal is not necessarily to lengthen life, but rather to ensure the best possible quality of life, which means, among other things, that a person remains independent for as long as possible.

Advertising and nutrition

1. Introduction

Everyone is free to eat and drink what they please, within certain limits. Unfortunately, however, choosing a healthy diet is not always easy and in order to make informed choices we need reliable information. Much of our information comes from advertising which obviously tends to be rather one-sided, and although as consumers we may be aware of its limitations, it can still manipulate and direct our choice of food.

Learning outcomes

After studying this chapter the student should be able to:
- describe the relationship between advertising and eating habits;
- offer examples of advertisements which are targeted at specific groups;
- understand how advertisements often generalise within an idealised situation;
- describe the function of the packaging of a food product.

2. Advertising food

Many millions of pounds are spent on advertising every year and, of that, 20% is spent on promoting foodstuffs and grocery products. In 1993, the cost of food advertising in the UK was £503 million. It is interesting to note that £102 million was spent on advertising sugar and confectionery but only £22 million was spent on advertising cereal products. Advertising, therefore, plays a very important role in the food supply industry and in the selection of food by the population at large.

One of the tasks of advertising is to convince people that a particular item is unique and to demonstrate how and why the purchaser can benefit from buying it.

Some advertising does this by talking about the product, but sometimes the product itself is barely mentioned and the class of people using it is highlighted instead, so that people who aspire to the lifestyle depicted in the advertisement will associate it with the product. For example, an advertisement may promote the idea of how choosing a particular brand of soft drink (whose advertising is aimed at young people) will mean that you are attractive, fashionable, and probably affluent. A brand of margarine will make your family happy and harmonious. A low fat spread will make you active and healthy; the right choice of coffee creates a cosy, romantic atmosphere. Sophisticated psychological techniques are used to appeal to the desires of the target audience and to mould their needs to the product, or even to create new needs where none existed before. In the midst of this, any analysis of the nutritional value of the product is normally minimal (if indeed present at all).

Advertising tries to make a link between a product and an ideal or desired situation.

For example: alcohol and cigarette advertising often conjures up a world of luxury, nostalgia is used in an advertisement where a certain brand of soup is associated with good old-fashioned values, or the tradition of a particular recipe is stressed. Some advertisements suggest that health or beauty will be yours if you use semi-skimmed dried milk or the right diet margarine on your bread. The image of women in advertisements is particularly significant. They tend to be beautiful, slim, feminine, and contented housewives and mothers. Advertisers try to make us believe that, if we use their products, we will function better as members of the family and of society.

Study activity 1

a. What do you think of the following statement? '
   "Through advertising, the food industry is creating a climate in which being overweight is considered a major social and psychological problem. The advertisers then take advantage of the anxiety and frustration involved, particularly that of women, in order to persuade people to buy low fat and 'light' products and various substitutes for meals."
b. Advertising costs a lot of money. Who pays for it?
c. What do you think of the following statement?: "Advertising must not be misleading but it is all right to exaggerate a little, as long as it is clear that it is an exaggeration."

3. Health and advertising

Since 1980, the use of terms like 'healthy' or 'good for your health' have been prohibited in advertising, because it is wrong to claim that any one food product is in itself healthy. A balanced diet depends on all the foodstuffs a person eats on a regular basis.

Advertising is, of course, intended to promote sales, so we tend to be given only information which emphasises the positive characteristics and advantages of the food product. For instance, the information on a yoghurt carton may inform you in large lettering that 'this product contains no artificial sweeteners', while you have to look much harder for the small text informing you it contains sugar. The labelling on a jar of peanut butter may state 'no colouring agents, flavour enhancers, or preservatives, but peanut butter does not contain these substances anyway.

Thus, statements referring to the health benefits of the product are actually designed to promote sales rather than health. Just think of pure vegetable cooking oil. The vegetable oils which are used as raw materials have been hardened through industrial processing and the product may contain a lot of the saturated fats which are associated with heart and arterial disease.

We can ask, of course, whether there is really any correlation between advertising and eating habits. The relationship between them is certainly very complex, but there is no doubt that advertising plays a part in our current excessive consumption of products like fat and sugar. Increasing consumption of snacks may also be attributable to advertising. The past few years have seen a huge growth in the range of savoury snacks and sweets, which we appear to need when watching television or having a drink.

4. Packaging

One function of food packaging is to protect the contents against damage, contamination, or drying out. It is also designed to promote sales. Most manufacturers believe that packaging should be pleasing to the eye and very often, attractive illustrations which bear little relation to the contents are shown. It is also common for more packing to be used than is required, and examples of double packaging (such as packet soup in a cardboard container) or extra large packaging (such as a box which is only half full) are easy to find.

All packaging costs money and is also environmentally harmful. In addition to the obvious waste of the earth's resources in the production of the packaging, every year we throw away millions of tons of packaging materials in the form of paper, cardboard, glass jars and bottles, aluminium cans, polythene and non-biodegradable plastic containers. Aiming to address this problem, local authorities have established more environmentally acceptable methods for collecting materials that can be recycled – glass, paper and sometimes plastic. An extension of the system of refundable deposits paid upon purchase of, for example, drinks in glass bottles, would also help to alleviate this problem. This is currently in use in only a few locations.

Study activity 2

Look at an advertisement or a TV commercial for a food product and answer the following questions:

a. What is the situation shown in the advertisement you selected? What do you think is the target group?
b. What is said about the actual product in the advertisement? Is anything said about the nutritional value?
c. Do you find this a responsible way to advertise? Explain your answer.
d. If the product you have selected is packaged, what do you think of the packaging?
e. Are you influenced by advertising? Explain your opinion.
f. Think of some packaged food products which could be sold in paper bags instead. Discuss the advantages and disadvantages of both methods.

5. Summary

Advertisers employ various techniques to promote sales. Advertising is often directed at specific groups of people, and tries to exploit existing needs or create new ones. Through advertising, we are led to believe that particular products can help us achieve certain ideals. This process costs a great deal of money, which ultimately comes from the consumer's pocket. The way in which advertising influences our choice of food is complex, but it undoubtedly contributes to our current excessive consumption of fat and sweet foods.

Final test for module 2

Instructions

This section consists of 90 statements. Each one may be correct or incorrect. The answer required is either YES or NO. In your assessment of whether the item is correct or not, you should base your decision only on the circumstances and facts given. The questions are arranged in groups, in the same order the related topics occurred in the text. After ensuring that all the questions have been answered, check the results of the test yourself using the answers at the back of the book.

1. A healthy diet will contain all the nutrients that the body needs and in the correct quantities.
2. A food product generally contains one particular nutrient.
3. Instant coffee is an example of a convenience food.
4. Milk is an example of a nutrient.
5. Carbohydrates and fats in the diet provide fuel for our body.
6. Proteins and minerals in the diet play an important part in structuring and restoring tissues.
7. A patient will always have a good nutritional status if his diet contains sufficient energy.
8. One characteristic of good nutritional status is that body weight and height are in proportion to each other.
9. Pale mucous membranes and fatigue can indicate poor nutritional status.
10. Malnutrition only occurs in the developing countries.
11. A diet with an excess of proteins, vitamins and minerals can have a negative influence on your health.
12. An unbalanced diet usually provides enough energy but contains too few nutrients.
13. Sometimes overweight people can suffer from malnutrition.
14. Because our bodies have a higher temperature than the environment, they constantly give off warmth. Warmth must therefore be continually produced for the body temperature to be maintained. This is why we need proteins.
15. Since 1950 we have started to consume more bread and less meat and cheese.
16. A lunch consists of wholemeal bread with margarine, cold meat and a glass of milk. This meal contains products from every group in the food guide.
17. All types of vegetables can adequately replace each other as far as the nutrients they contain are concerned.
18. On average, we consume some 8-10 kilos of sugar per person per year.
19. Sausages are in section four of the food guide.
20. Peanut butter is in section two of the food guide.
21. Through the **Food and Safety Act** standards can be set for the quality of foodstuffs.
22. The 'use before' date of a food product may be two days past before the product must be taken off the shelf.

23. If the quality of a recently purchased food product is not up to standard, you can complain to the Environmental Health Department.
24. The following foodstuffs are found in the food guide: potatoes, tomatoes, Edam cheese, corn oil, chicken, fish.
25. A preservative is an example of an additive which can be found in foodstuffs.
26. Additives in food are often simply cosmetic, to give the product a more pleasant outward appearance.
27. The small letter 'e' on the packaging indicates that there is an additive in the product.
28. After the digestive process, starch from bread is absorbed into the blood in the form of glucose.
29. Dietary fibre can be absorbed into the blood in the last part of the large intestine.
30. Fats can only be digested properly with the assistance of bile.
31. The amount of energy you need per day depends on, amongst other things, age, gender and appetite.
32. One gram of fat provides 38 kJ.
33. The elderly require less energy in their diet, because they have a higher metabolic rate and often undertake less physical activity.
34. If you consume more energy in your diet than you use, your body weight will increase.
35. Starch is found in bread, potatoes and pulses.
36. A glass of fruit juice (150 ml) contains an amount of sugar equal to six sugar cubes.
37. Foodstuffs rich in fat may contain vitamins A and D.
38. Salad oil and diet margarine can raise the cholesterol level in the blood.
39. Saturated fats are found in all hard margarines and butter.
40. Buttermilk and low fat yoghurt contain very little or no fat.
41. Mayonnaise contains as much fat as butter.
42. Mayonnaise contains a lot of unsaturated fats, whilst butter contains a lot of saturated fats.
43. An excess of proteins in the diet has a negative effect on the heart and arteries.
44. A low protein diet can eventually lead to anaemia, slow healing of wounds and lower resistance to infections.
45. You need meat every day.
46. The body consists of 50% water.
47. Drowsiness, listlessness and fatigue may be symptoms of dehydration.
48. Most people need extra vitamin preparations when there is an 'r' in the month.
49. Dietary fibre can be digested in the body.
50. Granulated sugar is necessary for the muscles.
51. Dietary fibre can be found in vegetable and animal foodstuffs.
52. Food with an extremely low fat content can cause deficiency of vitamins A and D.
53. Full fat milk and fatty meat contain saturated fats.
54. Cholesterol is a substance which is not necessary to the body.
55. Our diet generally lacks protein.
56. A fluid loss of 25% can be fatal.
57. People who do not get enough sunlight risk vitamin A deficiency.
58. Bleeding gums can indicate a vitamin C deficiency.
59. Children who consume a lot of sugar or sweet food run the risk of vitamin B_1 deficiency.
60. A serious lack of calcium and vitamin D can cause rickets.
61. Iodine plays a part in blood coagulation.
62. Iron is necessary for the formation of haemoglobin.
63. Milk contains a lot of iron.
64. There is a lot of iron in brown bread, green vegetables, and cheese.
65. People with high blood pressure are often advised to follow a low sodium diet.

66. Vitamin A is primarily found in animal foodstuffs rich in fat, and carotene is found in vegetable products.
67. Vitamin D helps you to see in the dark.
68. Sufficient quantities of vitamin C and iron in the diet will help to prevent anaemia.
69. Vitamin D promotes the formation of strong bones.
70. Mother's milk contains antibodies.
71. One example of a humanised formula is a mixture of cow's milk and water.
72. Green beans are vegetables rich in nitrate.
73. An infant of 8 months should be fed bottle or breast milk, one bowl of porridge, one bread-based meal and a hot meal per day
74. Boys usually mature more quickly than girls.
75. Toxoplasmosis can occur after eating roast beef.
76. PCBs are not transferred to mother's milk.
77. Aniseed, dill, and brown ale are reputed to 'stimulate' the production of mother's milk.
78. The elderly often suffer from constipation.
79. A meal rich in fat is often more difficult for the elderly to digest than it is for young adults.
80. The older one gets, the less one needs vegetables and fruit.
81. To slow down the process of bone de-calcification as much as possible, one requires a diet with sufficient milk and dairy products as well as physical outdoor exercise.
82. The following foodstuffs contain vitamin D: margarine, egg yolk and full fat yoghurt.
83. A cup of tea half an hour before a meal can usually stimulate the appetite.
84. Chewing problems can be caused by a deterioration of the teeth or poorly fitted dentures.
85. The elderly lose more fluid through the skin because their skin has become thinner.
86. An elderly person must take one litre of fluids a day.
87. An elderly person will be eating enough fruit if he has an orange every second day.
88. Schemes which provide hot meals for the elderly often help them to maintain their independence.
89. The main purpose of advertising is to promote sales.
90. In order to reach the consumer, the advertiser tries to identify the product with his or her lifestyle.

References and further reading

Black A and Rayner M, (1992) *Just Read the label: Understanding Nutrition Information in Numeric, Verbal and Graphic Formats.* HMSO, London.

Briony T, (ed), (1994) *Manual of Dietetic Practice.*2nd ed. Oxford/Blackwell Scientific Publications, Oxford.

British Nutrition Foundation, (1990) *Nutrition Labelling. Briefing Paper No. 21.* BNF, London.

Committee on Medical Aspects of Food Policy, (COMA), (1992) *Annual Report.* Department of Health, London.

Debry G, Bleyer R and Martin J M, (1977) Nutrition of the elderly. *Journal of Human Nutrition,* 31, 63-83.

Department of Health, (1988) *Present Day Practice in Infant Feeding.* HMSO, London.

Department of Health, (1989) *The Diets of British School Children.* HMSO, London.

Department of Health, (1994) *Eat Well. An Action Plan from the Nutrition Task Force to Achieve the Health of the Nation Targets on Diet and Nutrition.* Department of Health, London.

Department of Health, (1992) *Health of the Nation: A Strategy for Health in England.* HMSO, London.

The Food Safety Act and You .A Guide for the Food Industry, (1990) HMSO, London

The Food Labelling Regulations,(1984) SI 1305, HMSO, London.

Goodinson SM, (1986) Assessment of nutritional status. *Nursing* 3, (7), 252-258.

Health and Welfare Canada, (1992), *Canada's Food Guide to Healthy Eating.* Ministry of Supply and Services, Ottawa.

Kirk S F L, (1990) Adequacy of meals served and consumed at a long stay hospital for the elderly. *Care of the Elderly,* 2, (2), 77-80.

Nutrition and Teenagers. Fact File no 5, (1992) National Dairy Council Nutrition Service.

Ministry of Agriculture, Fisheries and Food, (1992) *Household Food Consumption and Expenditure 1991. Annual Report of the National Food Survey Committee.* HMSO, London.

Royal College of Midwives, (1992) *Your First Baby.* HHL Publishing, London.

Royal College of Midwives, (1991) *Successful Breastfeeding* (2nd ed) Churchill Livingstone, Edinburgh.

Scotland's Health: A Challenge to Us All *The Scottish Diet* (1993). *Report of a Working Party to the* Chief Medical Officer for Scotland. Scottish Office Home and Health Department, Edinburgh.

Steen B ,(1985) *Nutrition.* in *Principles and Practice of Geriatric Medicine,* Pathy M (ed.), John Wiley & Sons, Chichester.

Module 3

NUTRITION AND HEALTH PROBLEMS OF TODAY

Introduction Module 3

In this module we will look at health problems, diseases, and conditions which occur far more often today than they did in the past. Some examples of these are heart and arterial disease, cancer, obesity, and constipation. Although these diseases cannot be attributed to any single cause, it is clear that our diet plays an important part in their occurrence. We will describe some changes in our eating habits which are desirable for the prevention of some of these health problems, and make recommendations for dietary improvements.

Eating disorders like anorexia nervosa and bulimia nervosa are often viewed as modern phenomena, caused by present-day society's preoccupation with slimness and the idea of slimness being synonymous with beauty. As a result, people are encouraged to follow all sorts of diets. This may indeed contribute to the occurrence of eating disorders. We will discuss briefly some of the characteristics of such disorders and methods of treatment for people with anorexia nervosa and bulimia nervosa.

We have seen how a lack or an excess of certain nutrients can cause disease. However, food can also endanger our health through infection with micro-organisms, or by the presence of harmful substances. We will discuss how food can become contaminated, which harmful substances can be found in food, what the consequences of these are, and how, in practice, we can try to prevent such contamination.

Obesity is considered to be an overriding problem by a lot of people. We will look at its causes and effects, psychological and social as well as physical, and investigate the practicalities and the myths of some of the therapies available.

Food and modern nutritional diseases

1. Introduction

In Module 2 we noted that illnesses caused by malnutrition are relatively rare in Western society today. Indeed, an unbalanced diet with an *excess* of certain nutrients can pose a greater risk to our health. Such excesses contribute to the occurrence of the common diseases of the Western world (by which we mean those diseases that result mainly from our increased affluence). This does not mean that these diseases never occurred in the past, but it does mean, however, that they have increased in correlation with the growth of affluence in Western society. Such diseases include heart and arterial disease and cancer. Our choice of food can greatly influence their occurrence, particularly if our diet contains too much fat and sugar, too little dietary fibre, or too much alcohol. Such eating habits (often combined with a lack of physical exercise, too much stress or smoking) form major risk factors for our health. In this chapter, we will examine the relationship between our diet and the diseases of the Western world.

Learning outcomes

After studying this chapter the student should be able to:
- summarise the relationship between diet and the common diseases of today;
- give 10 recommendations for changes to improve our current eating habits;
- explain how five of these recommendations are important for the prevention of heart and arterial disease and provide practical advice for each recommendation;
- state which three recommendations are important for the prevention of cancer;
- name five diseases which are related to a lack of dietary fibre;
- state which two dietary recommendations are important for the prevention of constipation and diverticulosis.

2. Recommendations for a healthy diet

Our diet has a great deal to do with our health. A suitably balanced diet can form a sound basis for maintaining or improving our health. The 10 recommendations for a healthy diet listed in Module 2 Chapter 2 apply to everyone. They give all the nutrients that the body needs to grow, repair itself, and to carry out vital metabolic processes. Following the recommendations can help to prevent nutritional deficiencies and, most importantly, reduce the occurrence of diseases related to the excesses of the Western diet.

3. Our diet and heart and arterial disease

Heart and arterial disease are the major causes of death in this country. Over the past 10 years, around 40% of all registered deaths were caused by this form of disease. The most common is arteriosclerosis which is caused by a process that affects the walls of the arteries and which can occur at an early age. This gradually causes the artery walls to thicken and harden, obstructing the flow of blood (Figure 3.1.2). Eventually, arteriosclerosis can lead to a heart attack or stroke (or in some cases brain haemorrhage). This happens when an artery is blocked to such an extent that an area of the heart or brain is no longer supplied with blood, with the result that the tissue of this deprived area then dies.

Figure 3.1.1
From Food and Your Heart, British Heart Foundation, London, 1992

Food, Cholesterol and Coronary Heart Disease

Worldwide studies have examined the links between various aspects of the food which people eat and the amount of coronary heart disease they suffer. Looking at all the evidence, there is a striking link between heart disease and the amount of fat in the diet, particularly saturated fat. As the proportion of saturated fat in the diet increases – so do deaths from heart disease.

A heart attack is the end result of a long, slow process. Gradually the arteries which supply the heart muscle become narrowed by a fatty substance called "atheroma". People who have high levels of cholesterol in their blood are more likely to have a heart attack or suffer with angina, particularly if they are cigarette smokers or have a raised level of blood pressure. At one time it was thought that the blood cholesterol level was mainly the result of the amount of cholesterol eaten in food (dietary cholesterol). But further research has shown that eating foods which contain a lot of fat, especially saturated fat, has a much greater effect in pushing up the blood cholesterol level than the dietary cholesterol. This is because most of the cholesterol in our blood is made from saturated fat by the liver.

The Department of Health set up a special committee to look at all the evidence about diet and heart disease and how it could be prevented.

It reported that by comparison with other countries, the British had exceptionally high saturated fat consumption, high blood cholesterol levels, and high death rates from coronary heart disease. Their strongest recommendations were that:

– the total amount of fat in the UK diet should be reduced

– the amount of saturated fat should be reduced

Their report* recommended that we should aim to get less than 35% of our energy from fat and less than half that amount should be from saturated fat. At the time of the report the average person consumed about 42% of their calories as fat and surveys in the 1980s have shown that this pattern has not changed very much.

At the same time they suggested that people might also benefit from increasing the amount of fibre-rich foods like bread, cereals, fruit and vegetables that they eat.

The amounts of salt, sugar and alcohol should also be controlled and obesity avoided through a combination of appropriate food intake and regular exercise.

*Report of the Committee on Medical Aspects of Food Policy: diet and cardiovascular disease (1984).

Figure 3.1.2
Arteriosclerosis

a. normal artery
b. arteriosclerosis
1. connective tissue layer
2. muscle layer
3. elastic tissue
4. intima (inner layer of the artery)
5. hardening
6. degeneration of the intima

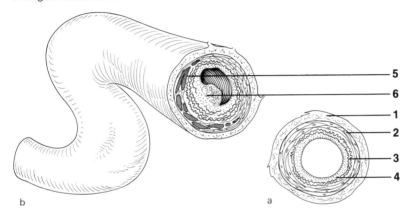

The causes of heart and arterial disease have not yet been precisely determined although a number of risk factors are known. The most important ones include a high cholesterol level in the blood, high blood pressure, smoking, lack of exercise and obesity. Seventy-five per cent of adult Scots have cholesterol levels above the acceptable range (<5.2 mmol/l). For around 1% of this total the cause is hereditary, but for the vast majority the increase is the result of lifestyle, including eating habits. The most important dietary recommendations for the prevention of heart and arterial disease are shown in Figure 3.1.3.

Study activity 1

a. Plan two three-course meals which meet the recommendations mentioned in Figure 3.1.3.
b. Which of the following foodstuffs contain a lot of saturated fat: walnuts, Cheddar cheese, packet margarine, sunflower oil, full cream milk, chocolate and peanut butter?

c. Give five examples of savoury sandwich fillings with minimal amounts of saturated fat.

Study activity 2

Mark is 35 years old and works in an office. His father, who is 68, was admitted to hospital for vascular surgery and, during one of his son's visits, it came out in conversation that heart and arterial disease had occurred in the family before. Two of his father's brothers also have heart problems. Although Mark feels physically fit, he worries about his health. He mentioned that he likes a cigar on the odd occasion and that he would not want to give this up. He would like to take a little more physical exercise and possibly change his eating habits, but he has no idea which foods would be more healthy for him. He asks you for practical advice.

a. What recommendations would you give? For each recommendation give three examples of foodstuffs he might try.
b. Mark likes fried food and has chips

Figure 3.1.3
Recommendations for a healthy heart

Recommended	Effect	Practical advice
avoid fat (particularly saturated fat)	reduces the risk of becoming obese – saturated fat can greatly increase the cholesterol level in the blood	use diet, low fat or non-fat margarine or spread on bread; use vegetable oil or soft margarine for cooking rather than animal fat or hard margarine; eat cottage or low fat cheese, rather than full fat cheese; avoid fatty meats; limit consumption of products with invisible fats like cakes, biscuits, crisps; eat no more than three eggs a week
use salt sparingly	less salt can lower the blood pressure	do not put salt, sauces, or other seasonings out on the table and use little salt or seasoning when cooking; avoid crisps, savoury snacks, sauces and tinned and packet soups; use a reduced sodium salt alternative
eat plenty of foods containing starch and dietary fibre	dietary fibre from vegetables, fruit, pulses and oatmeal products and an increase in starch foods contribute to the reduction of the cholesterol level in the blood;	eat plenty of bread, especially brown and wholemeal bread with a high fibre content (see the wrapping for the nutritional information); eat plenty of fruit, vegetables, pulses, legumes, porridge and other cereal products
attain and maintain your ideal body weight	obesity increases the risk of heart and arterial disease	eat less fat and sugar; drink less alcohol
drink at least three pints of fluid a day but drink alcohol only in moderation	too much alcohol raises the blood pressure and can cause obesity, thus increasing the risk of heart and arterial disease	do not get into the habit of having alcoholic drinks every day or having a great deal to drink on a regular basis, for instance, every weekend; when you do drink alcohol, limit your intake to, say, three glasses of wine or the equivalent in beer and spirits

with most meals. What is your opinion of this?

c. Mark's father likes to have a tasty snack at night, such as a few biscuits and cheese or a packet of crisps. His son occasionally brings him such snacks on his hospital visits. Do you think this is a good idea? Can you suggest a few healthier alternatives?

4. Our diet and the occurrence of cancer

After heart and arterial disease, cancer is the next most prevalent cause of death in this country, and the mortality rate due to cancer is constantly increasing. This is partly attributed to the fact that people are living longer than they used to, but research has shown that various factors can play a role. It is estimated that approximately 80% of all cancer cases are due to environmental factors, so prevention can play a vital role, and, although a lot is still unknown about the precise relationship between diet and cancer, there does appear to be a strong link between the two. Deficiencies in dietary fibre, vitamins A, C, E or selenium may be a factor in the development of certain types of cancer. These deficiencies can be avoided through a varied diet, which includes lots of fresh vegetables, fresh fruit and wholemeal products.

A EU body of cancer experts has devised a 'cancer code' for Europeans which provides guidelines for preventive action against cancer, or to assist in speedy diagnosis when it does occur.

The European Code Against Cancer

1. Do not smoke. If you do, stop as quickly as possible and certainly do not smoke in the presence of others.
2. Drink alcohol in moderation.
3. Be aware of the harmful effects of the sun.
4. Observe health and safety regulations at work, particularly when working with substances which can cause cancer.
5. Eat plenty of fruit, vegetables and cereal products which are rich in dietary fibre.
6 Avoid being overweight and do not eat too much fatty food.
7. Consult your GP:
    – if a mole changes shape or colour;
    – if you discover a lump or swelling;
    – if you have any abnormal bleeding.
8. See your GP if minor ailments such as coughing or hoarseness become persistent, if your bowel habits change or if there is inexplicable weight loss.
9. Have a cervical smear test carried out regularly.
10. Check your breasts regularly. If you are 50 years of age or older then you should undergo regular breast-screening.

A diet rich in fat increases the risk of cancer of the colon, prostate, and breast. Black patches can occur on foodstuffs when roasting, grilling, baking or barbecuing; these black patches may contain carcinogenic (cancer-causing) substances and, though risks are only slight, it is safer to eliminate them from the diet. For the same reason, frequent consumption of smoked food is not recommended.

Study activity 3

a. Which dietary recommendations are important in reducing the risk of cancer?

b. Suggest two examples of meals which comply with these recommendations.

Figure 3.1.4
Diverticula

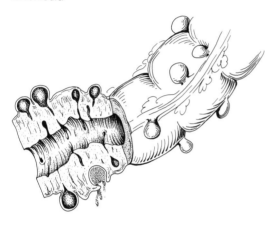

5. Our diet and constipation

Constipation is a common ailment. Related complaints include feeling bloated, wind, a rumbling stomach, cramps, bad breath, nausea, and headaches. A prime cause of constipation is a lack of dietary fibre. (As noted in Module 2, Chapter 3, dietary fibre has a laxative effect.)

In addition to constipation, lack of dietary fibre can cause diverticulosis, a disorder of the large intestine in which sacs form in the intestinal lining (Figure 3.1.4). A lack of dietary fibre and fluid can cause the faeces to be hard and dry, and this leads to exertion and straining on going to the toilet, creating high pressure in the intestines and aiding the development of sacs (diverticula). Diverticulosis occurs quite frequently among the elderly, and its symptoms commonly include a rumbling stomach, wind, stomach cramps, and a defecation pattern which alternates between constipation and diarrhoea. In addition, food residue can collect in the sacs, eventually leading to infection (this is then called *diverticulitis*). A diet with poor dietary fibre content is also related to cancer of the colon, haemorrhoids, and appendicitis.

Some foods which have been shown to be effective in the prevention of constipation, diverticulosis, cancer of the colon, haemorrhoids and appendicitis are listed in Figure 3.1.5

Figure 3.1.5
Recommendations for avoiding constipation

Recommended	Effect	Examples
eat plenty of dietary fibre	laxative effect	wholemeal bread, fresh vegetables, fruit, brown rice, wholewheat cereals, wholewheat pasta, pulses such as lentils, split peas, chickpeas
drink at least three pints of fluid a day	moistens stools	drink at least 10 glasses of liquid throughout the day

Study activity 4

a. Why is diverticulosis so common in Western Europe?

b. What relationship is there between dietary fibre and constipation?

c. List as many types of pulses and legumes as you can.

d. A 68-year-old man is in the neurological ward of a hospital. He sometimes suffers from constipation and he is hardly ever thirsty. Staff in the department have agreed that his fluid intake should be increased, but how should they approach the problem? What is more appropriate – freshly squeezed orange juice, or a whole orange? Why? What other dietary means would help to resolve the problem?

e. What is bran?

6. Summary

Diseases related to our diet may be influenced by various factors. This chapter discussed how eating habits can play a role in the occurrence of heart and arterial disease, cancer and constipation. A diet which contains too much energy, fat, sugar, salt, and alcohol, and too little dietary fibre poses a threat to health. We have also discussed 10 recommendations which can contribute to the prevention of cancer.

Eating disorders: anorexia nervosa and bulimia nervosa

1. Introduction

In developing countries where food shortages are common, obesity in men and women is often considered attractive. Elsewhere, however, being slim seems to be the ideal. Advertisers frequently confront us with images of thin people who are happy and affluent, and this greatly contributes to the idea that a slim body is the solution to all problems.

Magazines offer a wide range of diets and promise guaranteed success. Such dieting is often the beginning of serious eating disorders. This exaggerated emphasis on low body weight appears to be partly responsible for the development of anorexia nervosa (where a person forces him or herself to eat very little) or bulimia nervosa (where a person indulges in bouts of compulsive overeating).

Learning outcomes

After studying this chapter the student should be able to:
- give a brief description of the eating disorders anorexia nervosa and bulimia nervosa;
- describe the differences and similarities between anorexia nervosa and bulimia nervosa, both in physical characteristics and in eating behaviour;
- indicate the two basic principles on which the treatment of anorexia nervosa is based;
- explain the basis of the treatment of bulimia nervosa.

2. Anorexia nervosa

Case study

Angela, 20 years old.
'It all started five years ago. I began dieting, because I had gained a few pounds during my holidays. At 53 kg (8 1/2 stones) I wasn't really overweight, but a friend said, "You'd better watch out, you'll start to look like your neighbour soon." My neighbour was 173 cm (5 ft 8 in) tall, weighing at least 90 kg (16 stones). It was that remark which prompted me to go on a diet and, to begin with, it was great! I lost weight and was amazed at how easy it was!

But I was never satisfied. I never thought I was thin enough. I started putting my fingers down my throat after I had eaten, to bring it all up again. I still went to school, but I couldn't concentrate very well. The only thing I cared about was losing weight and getting thin. I was proud of that and it gave me a feeling of being in control and especially being in control of my body. I was constantly counting the calories in every mouthful of food. I started an intensive physical exercise programme as well. I would cycle for long distances, walk miles every day and I went jogging a lot as well. I continued losing weight, and even when I weighed 44 kg (7 stones), I still felt too fat. I even started to take large quantities of laxatives to keep losing weight.

At one point, my parents sent me to the doctor because they could see that something was wrong, but when I was there I made up a whole lot of other ailments and I didn't tell the doctor about my eating habits.

It wasn't until I was 18 that they found out that I had anorexia nervosa. I was admitted to hospital because I only weighed 38 kg (6 stones). While I was in the hospital I gained quite a lot of weight, mostly because I could eat more without loss of control. After I was discharged things went wrong again.

Some time later a friend put me in contact with a psychologist, and through the discussions I had with him I slowly started to understand the underlying problems. He arranged for me to join a group for people with eating problems and it was then that I realised that I wasn't the only one with an eating disorder. The group discussions helped me a lot. I discovered that I wasn't very satisfied with myself although I'm slowly figuring it out now. I have to learn to have self-respect, regardless of my weight. I'm slowly getting there.'

Study activity 1

a. Why do you think Angela was so proud of her great weight loss?
b. Why did Angela indulge in so much physical exercise?

c. Why would the support group have such a positive influence on her?

a. The occurrence of anorexia nervosa
Anorexia nervosa occurs mainly among females between the ages of 14 and 25, but there are also patients as old as 66. Only around 10% of the anorexia nervosa patients are male. This illness carries a high mortality rate in that 15% of patients eventually starve themselves to death. There is a new concern focusing on the increasing prevalence in schoolchildren.

b. Characteristics of anorexia nervosa
Anorexia nervosa involves an obsessive refusal of food, partly related to a desire to lose weight and an exaggerated fear of gaining weight. There are usually complex psychological causes underlying these fears. One common characteristic of anorexia nervosa patients is an inability to accept failure. They either want to do something perfectly, or not at all and they live in continual fear of failure. People with anorexia nervosa have no perception of their illness, and always feel that they are too fat, even if their weight is normal or below normal. They often lose 25% or more of their original body weight and particularly avoid foods which are rich in carbohydrates and fat. Their very limited food intake may be accompanied by vomiting and the use of laxatives.

A lot of anorexia nervosa patients take a surprising amount of physical exercise (they may seem to have endless stamina) and about 40% indulge in eating binges (bulimia). If an anorexic patient's body weight falls below a certain level, menstruation stops, but this can be artificially maintained by the use of the contraceptive pill.

Although anorexia nervosa patients compulsively refuse to eat, their thoughts are often dominated by food. For example, they often know exactly how many calories different foods contain. It is also common for an anorexic to cook a lavish meal for someone else, and yet not to take a single bite of it herself!

Figure 3.2.1
© The Guardian, 24/6/94

Anorexic twin finds road to recovery in Canada clinic

Angella Johnson

ANOREXIC sufferer Samantha Kendall, whose weight fell to 4 $^1/_2$ stone as a result of the disease which killed her twin sister, is recovering at a clinic in Canada.

Samantha, aged 27, from Birmingham, was admitted three weeks ago after she discharged herself from Solihull Hospital in the West Midlands to travel to the Montreux Counselling Centre in Victoria, British Columbia, which specialises in eating disorders.

It may take months, but Samantha is hopeful of beating her anorexia. "I grew up thinking I was a failure in everything. Now, I'm trying to accept that I, Samantha Kendall, am worth living for. And perhaps I am," she said.

The clinic concentrates on emotional care rather than weight gain. Even now, Samantha prefers not to know her true weight.

"My anorexic self will take over and tell me I'm selfish for enjoying myself. It will tell me I'm a fat pig for eating today and tell me I'm not worthy enough for good things."

Anorexia struck when she and Michaela were both 13.

"We just started comparing diets and copying each other," Samantha said. "People had always gone on about how fat we were."

On April 20 this year, Michaela died after collapsing at home.

3. Bulimia nervosa

Case study

Sarah (18 years old)
'It started last year. I was living on my own for the first time and I thought I would take full advantage of my freedom. I spent a lot of time with my classmates, who were mostly slimmer than me, and after a few jokes about my weight I decided to go on a diet. In the beginning everything went fine and people paid me compliments on my figure. But then hunger pangs began to abound, especially when I was alone in my room at night and was nervous or a bit fed up. Then I would get the feeling I had to compensate for something; I'd go to the kitchen and eat everything in the refrigerator, and then I'd go looking for sweets. I'd search all the cupboards for food - it didn't matter what I ate, as long as it filled me up. A whole packet of biscuits, bread with butter and jam, meat, cheese, a whole cake, a bar of chocolate, crisps, soft drinks, yesterday's leftovers - I'd eat anything I could

lay my hands on. Then I'd feel sick, and very guilty. The following day I would still feel ill and guilty so I would go on a strict diet. But the eating binges continued becoming a type of addiction. I didn't dare discuss it with anybody because I was so ashamed. The alternating pattern of eating binges and then strict dieting kept my weight at a reasonable level, but I was disgusted with my body and my eating behaviour, and that constantly put me in a bad mood.'

a. Occurrence of bulimia nervosa
Bulimia nervosa occurs in around 40% of anorexia nervosa sufferers, and it is also found in about 40% of people who are overweight. The eating binges are usually associated with vomiting, use of laxatives, or a period of fasting. Although bulimia occurs in both men and women, particularly between the ages of 15 and 35, it is mainly women who suffer from it. A lot of people react to a vague description of bulimia with comments like: 'Oh yes, I have the same problem. I can't keep my hands off crisps and biscuits either!' But

bulimia is quite different from simply eating too much because you enjoy it.

b. The characteristics of bulimia nervosa

Sufferers from bulimia nervosa consume large quantities of food in short periods of time, usually without even enjoying it. The frequency of these eating binges can range from a few times a month to several times a day and, during one such session a bulimic may eat a sufficient amount of food to maintain a person in food for several days. The food is often rich in energy and easy to eat, and this compulsive overeating is seldom noticed by other people as it usually takes place when the bulimic is alone. Bulimics are usually secretive about their eating because they are ashamed of it and the following example is typical.

Case study

A woman suffering from bulimia nervosa always tried to ensure that her husband was out of the house very early in the morning - long before he was due to leave for work. This enabled her to give in to her uncontrollable desire to eat privately and undisturbed. When her husband accused her of having an affair, she did not tell him the truth as she preferred to be accused of adultery rather than gluttony.

Bulimics will wolf down food usually without even tasting it and only after large quantities have been consumed is there a feeling of satisfaction. The compulsive overeating usually ends with vomiting, and there is an alternating pattern of fasting and excessive eating. Bulimics realise that their eating behaviour is abnormal and, after eating binges they often feel depressed and guilty. The binged food is usually 'junk food' and most often chocolate. The victims associate the food with guilt and have to vomit to rid themselves of the guilt. Their weight, nevertheless, is usually normal or slightly overweight.

Study activity 2

Make a chart showing the differences and similarities between people suffering from anorexia nervosa and those people suffering from bulimia nervosa. Pay particular attention to the physical characteristics and the eating behaviours which occur in each disorder.

4. Treatment for anorexia nervosa and bulimia nervosa

Every anorexia nervosa or bulimia nervosa sufferer should realise that the illness can be completely cured - provided that the motivation is there to get better.

The treatment for anorexia nervosa is founded on two basic principles: firstly, that the psychosocial problems underlying the illness should be dealt with; and secondly, that the patient's weight should be gradually increased. Where there is a serious degree of malnutrition, it will be necessary to admit the patient into hospital. For the most part, however, it is usually quite possible to treat anorexia nervosa sufferers on an out-patient basis using, for example, a team consisting of a doctor, a psychologist, and a dietitian.

Various types of therapy can be applied but, in general, the therapy will be more successful if attention is focused on the individual and his or her particular problems, rather than on weight gain. The usual approach is to use a behaviour treatment programme in which the patient is removed from the varying degrees of control of eating and other aspects of life, and responsibilities are gradually given back as a reward for progress in treatment (usually measured by weight gain).

The treatment of bulimia nervosa is also aimed at dealing with psychosocial problems, but additional support can be given through dietary recommendations. For example, the patient can be advised not to fast between eating binges but to follow a healthy and balanced diet. The patient may also be advised to eat an energy-rich snack shortly before the time at which an eating binge normally occurs. This encourages the bulimic patient to accept the overeating sessions and to learn gradually to enjoy what he or she is eating.

During therapy for bulimia, patients should be encouraged, through discussion, to understand the background of their eating behaviour, learn to accept their bodies and how to deal with food. They should be encouraged to enjoy food, to develop an awareness of their emotions, and to find a better form of expressing them rather than 'swallowing' them or 'spitting' them out.

Patients suffering from anorexia nervosa or bulimia nervosa are often admitted to hospitals or nursing homes and they require a lot of support and understanding. To simply eat regularly is difficult for them. Their fear of losing control over their eating behaviour is very real, and if staff take this fear seriously it can be of enormous help to the patients. Local support groups organised by hospitals specialising in eating disorders are also very valuable.

Information can be obtained from the Eating Disorders Association, Sackville Place, 44 Magdalen Street, Norwich, Norfolk. Telephone (0603) 621414.

5. Summary

Two eating disorders have been discussed in this chapter, anorexia nervosa and bulimia nervosa. These are often thought to be products of modern Western society. Anorexics strive to eat as little as possible, whereas bulimics regularly indulge in compulsive overeating. Both eating disorders are more common among women than among men and among young rather than older women. We have discussed the physical characteristics and the eating behaviours typical of each, and we have looked at some methods of treatment. Learning to eat regularly is very difficult for people with these disorders as is the successful implementation of treatment. A great deal of attention must be paid to the psychosocial aspects of the treatment, and the medical and nursing staff need to offer generous amounts of support and understanding.

Diet and safe food

1. Introduction

Stories about dangers in our food feature regularly in the media. It may be said, for instance, that certain foods contain excessive amounts of radioactivity, bacteria, hormones, pesticide residues or heavy metals like lead and cadmium. In this chapter, we will discuss numbers 8 and 9 of the 10 recommendations for a healthy diet that were listed in Module 2, Chapter 2. Most of the chapter will be concerned with food safety as regards the presence of micro-organisms, in particular the pathogenic bacteria (i.e. those causing disease), which are responsible for food infection or food poisoning. Every year, many thousands of people are victims of food infection or food poisoning. Common symptoms include nausea, vomiting, stomach cramps, diarrhoea, and sometimes headaches and fever. These symptoms are not always recognised as indications of food poisoning because often a 'stomach bug' is blamed for their sudden onset. However, in a great number of cases, food poisoning is the cause.

Most cases appear to originate in places where food is prepared for immediate consumption, such as the home, the kitchens of nursing homes and hospitals, shops and various catering establishments. Ready-made foods present particular problems (see Figure 3.3.1). Insufficient cooking or failure to heat food through to the correct temperature during preparation often causes contamination. Unrefrigerated storage in particular is often the cause of food infections or food poisoning. The people most at risk are the groups who are generally vulnerable, notably infants and the elderly. People with poor nutritional status due to some chronic illness or condition will also be more susceptible. In this chapter we will also explore ways of dealing with the presence of harmful substances in food.

Learning outcomes

After studying this chapter the student should be able to:
- describe in his or her own words the difference, in both causes and symptoms, between food infection and food poisoning;

- name the groups which are particularly susceptible to food poisoning or infection;
- explain why someone with poor nutritional status is at greater risk from food poisoning;
- list several foodstuffs which can spoil quickly;
- describe two situations which are ideal for the multiplication of bacteria and four situations which can slow down or prevent multiplication;
- list measures for preventing the contamination of food by bacteria and offer guidelines to prevent any bacteria that are already in food from multiplying;
- give examples of harmful substances which may be present, either by accident or naturally, in food;
- give practical recommendations to reduce the amount of harmful substances in food.

Study activity 1

Why do you think someone with poor nutritional status runs a greater risk of suffering from food poisoning?

Case study 1

Lunch in a nursing home consisted of the following courses: chicken soup, mashed potatoes with meatballs in gravy, green beans and pears with chocolate pudding. The meal was eaten by 49 elderly residents, 4 staff and 66 elderly people who had the hot meals delivered to their homes. Unfortunately, this meal was not as nice as it seemed.

Early that evening, one man in the nursing home began to suffer from diarrhoea. As the night progressed, more people fell victim to diarrhoea, symptoms of dehydration and shock. In total, 109 of the 119 people who had eaten the meal fell ill, and before the weekend was over 7 of them had died. The average age of those who died was 76. High levels of bacteria were found in the faeces of these people and an investigation concluded that the hand-rolled meatballs were the source of the infection. They had been insufficiently cooked during preparation. With a greater awareness of food hygiene, this outbreak of infection could have been prevented.

Case study 2

In a large hospital, an elderly woman died and 60 other people became ill as the result of food infection. Their symptoms included high fever and severe diarrhoea, and some of the older patients had to be put on a drip for several days to prevent dehydration. Tests carried out on the faeces indicated a bacterial infection. 'Toad-in-the-hole' which had been on the menu the previous day turned out to be the cause of this food infection.

2. Food infection and food poisoning

In practice, *food infection* is often called *food poisoning* even though there is a distinct difference between the two.

Food infection occurs as a result of the presence of a great number of bacteria in the food. About 12 hours after eating the infected food, stomach cramps and diarrhoea occur. Large amounts of bacteria may be found in food which has been insufficiently cooked or in food that has been improperly stored. In favourable conditions (30-40°C), one bacterium can multiply into 16 million bacteria within eight hours (Figure 3.3.2). If food containing such a number of bacteria is eaten, illness will almost certainly result.

Food poisoning is caused by toxins (poisonous substances) produced by bacteria. The symptoms, which occur quite rapidly (usually within 8 hours) after eating the contaminated food, commonly include nausea and vomiting. One type of bacterium which produces these toxins is often found in the nose and throat of healthy people, and in pus which is, for instance, found in boils or infected wounds. Toxins cannot be destroyed by heating,

and there is, therefore, no point in cooking food which has developed mould (such as fruit preserve and jam). Nor is removing the mould of any use, as the toxins may have already spread throughout the product.

Food infection and food poisoning are both easy to recognise. In many cases, two or more people will become ill at the same time with the same symptoms.

Figure 3.3.1
© The Herald 24/5/94

Child's death linked to food poisoning

by Margaret Vaughan

The toll of the West Lothian food poisoning outbreak yesterday rose to 42, mostly children, including the brother of a toddler who died last week.

The procurator-fiscal confirmed the death of two-year-old Clare Davison is being linked to the outbreak, thought to have been caused by contaminated milk.

Her brother Paul is one of four children reported to be seriously ill in Edinburgh's Sick Children's Hospital following the outbreak.

An 11-year-old boy remains on renal dialysis after his kidneys failed and a three-year-old girl was transferred to the hospital for specialist treatment. other victims are being treated at the City Hospital, St John's Livingston, or at home.

Environmental health officers were still taking samples from The Redhouse Dairy, at Blackburn in West Lothian, which has been closed.

A Lothian Health spokesman said it is increasingly likely the source of the outbreak was the dairy but the results of detailed tests being conducted at the Western General microbiological laboratories were still awaited.

Of the 42 people now suffering the symptoms of food poisoning – 32 children and 10 adults – there was confirmation that, so far, 23 had been attributed to the E-coli 0 157 bacterium.

It emerged yesterday there was an outbreak of E-coli 0 157 in Fife last month, which struck down 10 people including an 18-month-old baby and two adolescents.

Dr Mike Roworth, a public health consultant for the region, said, in that case, contaminated meat sold from a butcher shop chain was implicated. The same consignment of contaminated meat was thought also to have been responsible for similar outbreaks in Lothian, Ayrshire, and Forth Valley.

The E-coli 0 157 organism lives in the gut of animals and is classically associated with beef

products, he added. It was rare to find contamination in milk which had been pasteurised.

"The difficulty is that it is difficult to isolate. It can be potentially lethal."

The organism produces a toxin, verocytoxin, which damages the lining of the bowel, causing bleeding. It can also cause a disorder of the blood, haemolytic uraemic syndrome, which leads to kidney failure, more common in young children than in adults.

At Ruchill Hospital in Glasgow, which co-ordinated reaction to the previous outbreak, public health specialist Dr Barbara Davies said what little evidence was available from West Lothian suggested the two outbreaks were not related.

Professor Michael Jackson of Strathclyde University's environmental health department said: "In previous cases, the food source has never been traced. It is generally associated with poor hygiene and contamination can occur through animal faeces or person to person spread."

Mr Hugh Annan, procurator-fiscal at Linlithgow, yesterday confirmed that Clare Davison's death at her Bathgate home last Thursday is being linked to the outbreak of food poisoning.

"Further tests are being carried out which could determine whether or not that is the case."

Mr Robert Haston, the owner of the dairy which has been closed, is co-operating fully with environmental health officers but did not wish to comment further.

In response to the criticism by West Lothian District Council of the way in which the public was informed of a potential health risk, a spokesman for Lothian Health Board said the timing of the first public statement had been decided jointly by members of the Lothian Outbreak Control team, which included staff from the council's own environmental health department.

Study activity 2

    a. In practice, how can you tell the difference between food infection and food poisoning?

    b. Why do you think fast-food outlets and restaurant kitchens are frequently inspected by the Environmental Health Inspectors?

    c. What might be a problem with the use of raw eggs in a pudding made in the kitchen of a nursing home or similar establishment?

3. How does food become contaminated?

Bacteria are present in every kitchen, no matter how hygienically it is maintained. Many foodstuffs and drinks form an excellent breeding ground for bacteria. Bacteria are found particularly predominantly in meat, meat products, fish, shellfish, dairy products, and pastries. If the bacteria do not find their way into the kitchen *in* the food, however, then people will *bring* them in. Nobody is free of bacteria.

Those bacteria that are most likely to cause disease and food spoilage multiply rapidly between the temperatures of 15 and 40°C, and the higher or lower the temperature gets outwith this range, the slower they multiply (Fig. 3.3.2). Bacteria are destroyed if the temperature rises above 60°C, as will happen during roasting, frying or boiling, and they multiply far less quickly in the refrigerator. They cannot multiply when they are deep-frozen, but they do stay alive, and when the food is defrosted bacteria start to multiply. If food is defrosted and then refrozen, the next time it is defrosted it is certain to contain a substantial colony of bacteria.

It should be noted that food which is contaminated does not always look as if it has 'gone off', and it may even taste and smell quite normal. Raw meat is always contaminated with pathogenic organisms, and mincing it spreads the bacteria through the meat, so products where minced meat has been used can spoil very quickly if they are not stored and prepared correctly. The bacteria present on raw products, such as meat and vegetables can also contaminate cutlery or kitchen utensils with which they come into contact. The water which thaws from frozen meat can also be a source of contamination.

Frequently, food is contaminated because it has been in contact with contaminated hands. It can also be infected with bacteria if it has not been heated to a high enough temperature, or for a long enough period of time. Bacteria do not survive easily in dry, sweet, salty, or acidic foods such as biscuits, jam, smoked bacon, or pickles.

Figure 3.3.2
Bacteria multiplication in relation to storage temperature and time

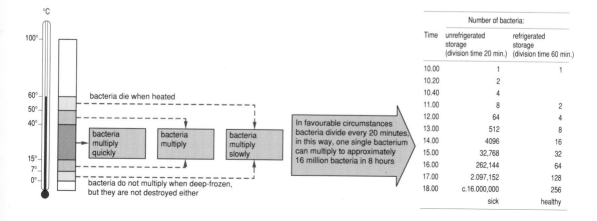

Time	Number of bacteria:	
	unrefrigerated storage (division time 20 min.)	refrigerated storage (division time 60 min.)
10.00	1	1
10.20	2	
10.40	4	
11.00	8	2
12.00	64	4
13.00	512	8
14.00	4096	16
15.00	32,768	32
16.00	262,144	64
17.00	2.097,152	128
18.00	c.16.000,000	256
	sick	healthy

In favourable circumstances, bacteria divide every 20 minutes; in this way, one single bacterium can multiply to approximately 16 million bacteria in 8 hours.

Figure 3.3.3
Which foods to keep where

Store the most perishable food in the coldest part of the fridge.

Coldest zone: 0°C to 5°C	Cool zones	Salad bin
Store here foods that must be kept cold to keep them safe. Wrap or cover all raw or uncooked foods	Store here foods that are best kept cool to help them stay fresher longer	This is the warmest part of the fridge
Examples Pre-cooked chilled foods e.g. ready meals, scotch eggs, pork pies; Soft cheeses; Cooked meats e.g. ham; Prepared salads (including pre-washed chopped, pre-packed mixed green salads, as well as rice salad, potato salad etc.); Desserts e.g. fromage frais; Home-prepared food and leftovers; Cream cakes	Examples Milk, yoghurt; Fruit juices; Hard cheeses e.g. cheddar; Opened jars and bottles of salad dressings, sauces, jams when labelled 'keep refrigerated'; Fats e.g. butter, margarine, low-fat spreads, cooking fats, lard; Eggs You can use special compartments if you have them.	Examples Vegetables, fruit, fresh salad items e.g. unwashed whole lettuce, whole tomatoes, radishes , etc.

Always keep raw meat, poultry and fish at the bottom of the fridge to stop them dripping on or touching other foods.

Even if pre-wrapped, put them in containers or extra wrapping to make quite sure.

Study activity 3

a. List a number of foodstuffs which spoil quickly.

b. Why does yoghurt not spoil as quickly as milk?

c. Why does mince always have to be heated especially thoroughly?

d. What can happen if raw meat and cooked meat are placed next to each other on a plate?

e. Describe the ideal circumstances for the multiplication of bacteria.

f. What circumstances can slow down or prevent the multiplication of bacteria in food?

g. What will spoil more quickly, jam, or low calorie jam? Why?

h. Why is it better to allow hot meals to cool down for a short while before refrigerating them?

4. The prevention of food poisoning and food infection

The most important measures for the prevention of food poisoning and infection are:
- food should be handled hygienically;
- it should be kept in cool storage (but not for too long);
- it should be cooled quickly and/or frozen.

The overview below gives some practical tips for preventing food contamination and the multiplication of bacteria.

Food is infected by bacteria as a result of:
- heating food at too low a temperature or for too short a time, thus allowing the contaminants to stay alive;
- touching food with contaminated hands;
- inadequate cleaning of utensils, chopping boards and sinks.

Contamination can be prevented by:
- minimum contact with food by the hands;
- washing the hands thoroughly after handling raw meat;

- using clean utensils to prepare food;
- thorough cleaning after use, of dishes, plates and chopping-boards which have been in contact with raw foodstuffs;
- avoiding the use of wooden spoons and ensuring thorough cleaning of sieves and graters;
- defrosting meat in a sizeable dish so that all the thawed water can be drained and the dish can then be washed in hot water;
- keeping raw food separate from cooked food;
- not storing dishes or pots containing food on the floor;
- covering food at all times;
- always heating mince thoroughly;
- when reheating food (whether in a conventional oven or in a microwave), always heat it thoroughly at a temperature of over 60°C;
- keeping insects out of the kitchen.

Bacteria will multiply most rapidly when:
- food is not refrigerated;
- meals prepared for later consumption are allowed to cool too slowly;
- pre-cooked meals are heated up too slowly;
- food is kept warm for a long time at too low a temperature.

To prevent bacteria from multiplying:
- always keep the temperature in the refrigerator below 7°C;
- do not put warm foodstuffs into the refrigerator;
- put perishable foodstuffs in the refrigerator as soon as possible after you have bought them;
- never keep leftovers for more than two days;
- do not prepare food too far in advance.

Study activity 4

a. Pre-cooked custard for an evening meal is delivered to a ward at 2 o'clock in the afternoon. This is immediately divided into individual portions. The custard is put in the microwave at 5 o'clock and then served hot. Why is this a poor procedure for serving the custard? Suggest a safer method.

b. In hospital, it is always extremely important to prevent food poisoning. List four measures for preventing the contamination of food by bacteria, then list four ways of preventing the bacteria in food from multiplying rapidly.

5. The presence of harmful substances in food

In addition to micro-organisms and their toxins, food can present a health risk through the presence of either pollutants or harmful substances which do not naturally occur in food but which contaminate it by accident. The micro-organisims may originate from industrial processes, exhaust fumes or household products and come into contact with the food through soil, air, or water. As a consequence of this contact the micro-organisms become absorbed and retained by plants or animals and are thus present in our food. Examples include traces of veterinary medication in meat, pesticide residues in vegetables, fruit and cereals, heavy metals (such as lead from exhaust fumes, cadmium from fertiliser, and mercury from waste products) in crops, and in offal such as liver and kidney, and even dioxin in mother's milk.

Levels of contaminants in our food are subjected to monitoring but their presence cannot always be prevented. Note that the risk of contaminants in food from animal sources is greater than the risk in food from vegetable sources. Because of their higher position in the food chain, animals absorb more contaminants in their food than do plants. Thus, the higher up in the food chain, the higher the concentration of contaminants. For instance, seals and birds of prey are at the top of their particular food chain, and they store the toxic substances in their fat reserves. In winter or while fasting, the fat reserves are used up, the

contaminants are released, and the harmful effect of these on the body is one reason why these animals tend to die more frequently in winter. The liver and kidney of farm animals often contain residues of veterinary medication or heavy metals and it is therefore better to avoid eating these foods too often. This also applies to freshwater fish and eels, which often have contaminants from water pollution stored in their fat tissue.

Food which is charred – during roasting, grilling or barbecuing, for example – may contain carcinogenic substances (particularly polycyclic hydrocarbons). It may, therefore, be wise to discard the black parts of such food. Carcinogenic substances are also formed when deep-frying fat is heated for a long time, and when it is heated to over 180°C especially when residues of the fried food remain in the fat.

Mould which has grown on food products can contain harmful toxic substances (toxins), though this does not apply where the mould has been added intentionally - as it is, for example, to certain blue cheeses. Once mould has grown, the toxins can spread throughout the product. Removal of only the mouldy portion does not, therefore, ensure that the rest of the food is free from toxins – it is better to discard the entire product.

One harmful substance which is found naturally in food is nitrate. Where there are high levels of nitrate, there is a risk that it will form nitrite, which is poisonous. This transformation can take place in the mouth and the gastrointestinal tract, but it may also take place in the food itself if it has been stored unrefrigerated for a long time, or when leftover vegetables rich in nitrate are reheated. Nitrite poisoning causes a lack of oxygen, and poses a particular threat to infants.

Nitrate is found naturally in vegetables and drinking water. Vegetables rich in nitrate include potatoes, endives, celery, Chinese leaves, beetroot, lettuce (except iceberg lettuce), spinach, and fennel. The use of fertilisers can greatly increase the nitrate level, and fresh greens which are supplied from greenhouses in the winter have a high level. Whilst this concern is acknowledged by some health agencies, such foods are not usually restricted.

There is a further potential problem with nitrite in that it binds with certain proteins in the stomach to form nitrosamines. Tests on laboratory animals have shown that nitrosamines have carcinogenic properties, and a meal which combines vegetables rich in nitrate with fish can significantly raise the level of nitrosamines in the gastric juices.

Solanine is another toxic substance found naturally in potatoes, particularly when they have gone green and have started to shoot. Removing the green parts and shoots reduces the solanine level. Boiling potatoes also reduces the level as solanine is transferred to the water and then poured away. Any form of heating will also partially destroy the solanine. Excessive quantities can lead to vomiting, diarrhoea and fainting. Such instances are rare and the amount of potatoes needed to be eaten would be something like 8 kg (17.5 lb) of potatoes at one sitting!

How can we eat safely?

- Keep the diet varied. All foods contain some beneficial and some harmful components, but by eating a wide range of foods the danger from any one is minimised;
- Eat more vegetables than food from animal sources;
- When eating vegetables and fruit, remove the peel or wash them thoroughly so that as much pesticide residue as possible is removed. Try to choose organic products which have been grown without the use of artificial fertiliser or pesticides;
- Try to avoid charred food by cutting off all the burnt bits;
- When deep-frying, do not heat the fat or oil above 180°C (the temperature at which the fat starts to smoke). Strain the fat or oil thoroughly after use and discard it as soon as it becomes dark-

coloured (so never top it up!);
- Throw away food such as fruit, bread, jam, fruit in syrup, peanuts and other nuts if there is any sign of mould. If cheese has only a small area of mould, cut away the affected part together with a generous part of the surrounding area, but if there is a lot of mould, throw away the whole piece of cheese;
- Remove shoots and any areas with green discoloration from potatoes and, preferably, cook them without the peel (as the peel is often treated with anti-sprouting pesticides), or else use organic potatoes.

Study activity 5

a. In your opinion, how great a risk is eating nitrates and nitrosamines?
b. Plan a one-day menu with three meals, and three between-meals snacks in which there are as few harmful substances as possible.

6. Summary

Every year thousands of people fall victim to food infection or food poisoning. Infants, the elderly, and people with a poor nutritional status are particularly susceptible. The differences in symptoms and causes between food poisoning and food infection have been described, and practical measures to minimise their risk have been discussed. An outline has been given of the sorts of harmful substances which may occur in food, either naturally or by contamination, and the chapter concluded with a list of guidelines for dealing with such substances.

Food and obesity

1. Introduction

The terms 'overweight', 'obesity', 'adiposity', and 'fat' are used if the body's mass of fat is proportionally too great. The cause of this seems simple: more food is taken in than the body needs. However, many factors may play a role in the development of obesity.

Today, in Western Europe, approximately one in every three people is keen to lose weight. Many consider themselves too heavy simply because their body weight is greater than the fashionable ideal. Any slight divergence from this notion of perfection is seen as a threat, even though there is no medical reason for concern. A huge variety of diet foods and special formulas for rapid weight loss promise success, but the slimming industry and advertisers are often the only ones who see any positive results.

In this chapter, we will look at the health risks and the psychological and social aspects of being overweight. We will also investigate the practicalities and the myths of some of the weight loss therapies available today.

Study activity 1

What is the point at which you think someone could be described as overweight?

Learning outcomes

After studying this chapter the student should be able to:
- explain the meanings of the terms 'overweight', 'obesity' and 'fat';
- describe two methods for determining a healthy body weight;
- list four possible causes for the development of obesity;
- make five dietary recommendations for the prevention of obesity;
- explain why a 'strict diet' seldom produces any results;
- describe the psychological, social and physical consequences of obesity;
- explain why the distribution of body fat has an important influence on health;
- evaluate slimming products and diets which promise slimness;

- make five recommendations for the treatment of obesity;
- list two objectives of a low energy or weight-reducing diet;
- list some foodstuffs which contain negligible amounts of energy, and which are therefore suitable for a low energy or weight-reducing diet;
- offer three tips for combating hunger pangs;
- explain why foodstuffs rich in dietary fibre are suitable for a low energy or weight-reducing diet.

2. The borderline between a healthy weight and obesity

There are two ways of estimating the healthy individual body weight, as follows:

a. The objective method

There are various tables which indicate the so-called 'ideal' weight. Some authorities recommend using the Quetelet Index (or Body Mass Index) method for determining the appropriate body weight. The Quetelet Index (QI) is calculated by dividing the weight in kilograms by the square of the height in metres. Thus,

$$QI = \frac{weight\ (kg)}{height^2\ (m)}$$

The higher the QI, or Body Mass Index (BMI), the greater the fat percentage in the body.

Case study

Anne weighs 66 kg and her height is 1.73 metres.

$$QI = \frac{66}{(1.73 \times 1.73)} = 22$$

A healthy body weight for both men and women is a QI between 19 and 25, so Anne's weight is fine.

A person with a QI of between 25 and 30 is moderately overweight (Grade I obesity), and one with a QI of 30 or more is seriously overweight (Grade II obesity). Anne, for instance, would be seriously overweight if she were to weigh 88 kg (Figure 3.4.1). According to this objective method, 4% of men and 6% of women are seriously overweight and it is estimated that 34% of men and 24% of women over 20 years old are moderately overweight.

Figure 3.4.1
Weight analysis based on the Quetelet Index (BMI)

Height	Healthy weight QI = 20	Moderately overweight QI = 25	Seriously overweight QI = 30
1.51 m	46 kg	57 kg	68 kg
1.54 m	47 kg	59 kg	71 kg
1.57 m	49 kg	62 kg	74 kg
1.60 m	51 kg	64 kg	77 kg
1.63 m	53 kg	66 kg	80 kg
1.66 m	55 kg	69 kg	83 kg
1.69 m	57 kg	71 kg	86 kg
1.72 m	59 kg	74 kg	89 kg
1.75 m	61 kg	77 kg	92 kg
1.78 m	63 kg	79 kg	95 kg
1.81 m	66 kg	82 kg	98 kg
1.84 m	68 kg	85 kg	102 kg
1.87 m	70 kg	87 kg	105 kg
1.90 m	72 kg	90 kg	108 kg
1.93 m	74 kg	93 kg	112 kg
1.96 m	77 kg	96 kg	115 kg

One drawback to this objective method of weight evaluation is that it makes no reference to how the individual feels about his or her weight. Moreover, a QI value of 25 or more does not necessarily indicate excessive fat reserves, it might be due to unusual muscle development, a heavy body framework or fluid retention in the tissue. However, a QI of over 30, with reasonable certainty, points to an excessive level of fat in the body.

Figure 3.4.2 Food and Your Heart, British Heart Foundation 1992 London

Keeping a Healthy Weight

For several health reasons, it's important to keep weight under control and by using the chart it is possible to see what is the ideal weight for a particular height. If it is necessary to lose some weight, then the tips given earlier for reducing fat intake will also help to reduce your calories. Some people still mistakenly believe that foods like bread and potatoes should be avoided in order to lose weight. But these can be helpful in producing a feeling of fullness and satisfaction while eating fewer calories because of the reduction of fat. It is also helpful to take more exercise, which helps to burn up calories as well as in-creasing the fitness of the heart. It's tempting to hope that special mixtures and fad diets will get rid of the problem of overweight quickly and painlessly. But these remedies usually only work in the short term and some may even be danger-ous. Ready-prepared, calorie-counted meals may be convenient and helpful but are not a real answer in view of the price and limited range of dishes. To lose weight and keep those extra pounds off, losing weight should always be a gradual process (one kilo/2lb per week) based on a low fat pattern of eating, and regular moderate exercise like brisk walking or climbing stairs.

Men weight without clothes (st)
add 6lb if you weigh yourself in your clothes

Height	Average Weight	Acceptable Weight Range	Obese
5ft 2in	8st 11lb	8st 0lb – 10st 1lb	12st 1lb
5ft 3in	9st 1lb	8st 3lb – 10st 4lb	12st 5lb
5ft 4in	9st 4lb	8st 6lb – 10st 8lb	12st 10lb
5ft 5in	9st 7lb	8st 9lb – 10st 12lb	13st 0lb
5ft 6in	9st 10lb	8st 12lb – 11st 2lb	13st 5lb
5ft 7in	10st 0lb	9st 2lb – 11st 7lb	13st 11lb
5ft 8in	10st 5lb	9st 6lb – 11st 12lb	14st 3lb
5ft 9in	10st 9lb	9st 10lb – 12st 2lb	14st 8lb
5ft 10in	10st 13lb	10st 0lb – 12st 6lb	14st 13lb
5ft 11in	11st 4lb	10st 4lb – 12st 11lb	15st 5lb
6ft 0in	11st 8lb	10st 8lb – 13st 2lb	15st 11lb
6ft 1in	11st 12lb	10st 12lb – 13st 7lb	16st 1lb
6ft 2in	12st 3lb	11st 2lb – 13st 12lb	16st 9lb
6ft 3in	12st 8lb	11st 6lb – 14st 3lb	17st 1lb
6ft 4in	12st 13lb	11st 10lb – 14st 8lb	17st 7lb

Women weight without clothes (st)
add 6lb if you weigh yourself in your clothes

Height	Average Weight	Acceptable Weight Range	Obese
4ft 10in	7st 4lb	6st 8lb – 8st 7lb	10st 3lb
4ft 11in	7st 6lb	6st 10lb – 8st 10lb	10st 6lb
5ft 0in	7st 9lb	6st 12lb – 8st 13lb	10st 10lb
5ft 1in	7st 12lb	7st 1lb – 9st 2lb	11st 0lb
5ft 2in	8st 1lb	7st 4lb – 9st 5lb	11st 3lb
5ft 3in	8st 4lb	7st 7lb – 9st 8lb	11st 7lb
5ft 4in	8st 8lb	7st 10lb – 9st 12lb	11st 12lb
5ft 5in	8st 11lb	7st 13lb – 10st 2lb	12st 2lb
5ft 6in	9st 2lb	8st 2lb – 10st 6lb	12st 7lb
5ft 7in	9st 6lb	8st 6lb – 10st 10lb	12st 12lb
5ft 8in	9st 10lb	8st 10lb – 11st 0lb	13st 3lb
5ft 9in	10st 0lb	9st 0lb – 11st 4lb	13st 8lb
5ft 10in	10st 4lb	9st 4lb – 11st 9lb	14st 0lb
5ft 11in	10st 8lb	9st 8lb – 12st 0lb	14st 6lb
6ft 0in	10st 12lb	9st 12lb – 12st 5lb	14st 12lb

b. The subjective method

The subjective method takes account of a person's own opinion of his or her weight. The ideal weight is the one at which they feel comfortable and content with their body. It may be difficult to be honest about this, of course, and people can be strongly influenced by friends, by advertising, or by fashion trends. In the latter two instances, models who radiate happiness, security, success, and wealth are almost always slim. These images encourage many people to try to lose weight.

These ideals change according to our culture and the time in which we live.

3. Why are people overweight?

Before a person tries to lose weight by any particular method, it is sensible to try to trace the possible causes of the obesity.

a. The direct cause

The direct cause of obesity is clear. More energy is consumed than the body uses. The excess energy is then stored in the form of fat. It is more useful to ask why this is happening, in other words, what are the indirect causes?

b. The indirect causes
Physical factors

Heredity probably has something to do with the occurrence of obesity, but the fact that there are a lot of overweight people in one family does not necessarily mean there is a hereditary predisposition. It is quite possible that their shared living and eating habits encourage obesity.

Obesity occasionally has metabolic causes, such as an underactive thyroid gland, and some medicines, such as prednisone and lithium, can cause a weight increase. Stopping smoking can also lead to weight gain in that food, and especially sweets, are used as a substitute for cigarettes.

Psychological factors

Psychological factors can greatly influence people's eating behaviour. Unpleasant experiences, for example, can depress the appetite in some people and yet stimulate it in others.

Three types of eating behaviour which may result in obesity can be distinguished:
- emotional eating, or eating as a reaction to stress (for example, eating to get rid of nerves or aggressive feelings in situations where expressing them is difficult or impossible);
- eating as a result of external stimuli; it is sometimes impossible to resist mouth-watering snacks;
- dieting - some people can actually gain weight by dieting, as can be seen in the example below.

Case study – *emotional eating*

'When I'm feeling down I always grab some goodies for comfort: a bar of chocolate, a bag of crisps, that type of thing. This is a habit I picked up when I was younger. I can still remember that I always got sweets or crisps from my mother if I had fallen down or if something unpleasant had happened.'
Ann (38 years old)

Case study – *gaining weight from dieting*

'I really wanted to lose 12 lbs before the summer, so I followed a diet I found in a magazine. It was a strict diet based on 500 kcal (2,100 kJ) a day, and it promised rapid weight loss. I couldn't stick to it though. I was always feeling weak and hungry, and after just a week temptation got the better of me. I feasted on chocolate and peanuts. This made me feel very guilty. Another diet I couldn't stick to! Out of frustration I started to eat even more, and I ended up weighing more after the diet than I did before.'
Margaret (45 years old)

The more strict the diet, the more difficult it is to stick to it. There will be a stronger inclination to break it and, if doing this results in a feeling of guilt, it may start off a vicious circle (Figure 3.4.3).

Figure 3.4.3
The vicious circle which may result from too strict a diet

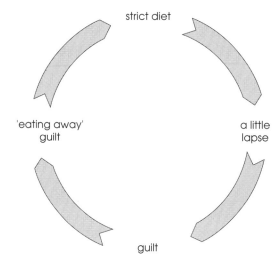

strict diet

'eating away'
guilt

a little
lapse

guilt

Social factors
Less healthy eating habits can be acquired at a young age, partly through parental influence. If, for example, children are forced to eat everything on their plate, they may end up eating more than they actually need.

Regular eating of sweets or savouries may also be due to habits which were acquired in childhood. Many parents misguidedly give their children sweets, chocolate, crisps, and sweet juice drinks just to keep them quiet or to stop them from whingeing. Such eating habits contribute to the very poor dental health which is found in British children and can become a fixed part of a person's lifestyle and thus contribute to obesity.

Study activity 2

What is your opinion of the following statements?:
- life is a lot easier if you are thin;
- it is more important for a woman to be thin than for a man;
- fat people have to become thin to start living;
- it is difficult to nurse overweight people;
- people can be pleasantly plump without being ugly.

Study activity 3

Think of some reasons why it is particularly women who often have problems with their weight.

4. The consequences of obesity

Obesity can bring with it health problems, both psychosocial and physical.

a. Psychosocial problems
Slimness seems to be the ideal, and this can cause overweight people to be discontented with their body and give them a negative self-image. As a result, being fat becomes a psychological burden and starts to influence the way in which the overweight person interacts with others. Sometimes overweight people try more or less to isolate themselves from contact with the outside world.

b. Physical consequences of obesity
In addition to the psychosocial problems, if a person is overweight there can also be physical health risks. In particular, seriously overweight people generally tend to be ill more often than those with a healthy body weight. Obesity increases the risk of developing diabetes mellitus, heart and arterial disease, high blood pressure, gout, problems affecting bones and joints, menstruation problems, varicose veins, shortness of breath, complications during surgery, hiatus hernia, and dermatosis.

In addition to the body weight itself, the distribution of fat over the body has important effects on our health. If the fat is primarily stored in the abdomen region there is an increased risk of diabetes mellitus, gout, hypertension, and heart and arterial disease. The larger the size of the waist, the greater the risk of such conditions occurring. This distribution of fat, commonly found in men, gives the body a typical apple shape. Women who are overweight often have fat on the hips and thighs, giving the body a pear shape. This latter type of fat distribution is more favourable. Research has shown that 'pear-shaped' people are less at risk from these conditions though they do have an increased risk of varicose veins.

A simple method for assessing the distribution of fat over the body is to calculate the waist-hip ratio. If this ratio is greater than 1 for a male, and 0.83 for a female, this signifies a surfeit of fat in the abdomen.

Study activity 4

a. Calculate your own hip-waist ratio.
b. What is the difference between medically overweight and being overweight according to fashion trends?

Figure 3.4.4
© The Telegraph 2/2/94

Slimmers' scent of success

by Roger Highfield, Science Editor

SMELLS could become a new weapon in the battle of the bulge. Evidence that hunger pangs can be alleviated with the help of apple, mint and banana odours has come from a pilot study carried out in America.

Over a six-month period, 3,193 subjects who were at least 10lb overweight inhaled a variety of scents three times in each nostril whenever they felt hungry. More than half of the patients – those who felt bad about overeating – lost around 5lb every month.

The study, by Dr Alan Hirsch of the Smell and Taste Treatment and Research Foundation, with Dr Ramon Gomez of the University of Illinois Medical School in Chicago, will be presented to smell researchers at a meeting in Florida in April.

In the pilot study, patients who had a poor ability to smell and showed other traits, such as eating more than five times a day and a dislike of chocolate, tended not to lose weight.

Dr Hirsch said it was possible the aversion to chocolate arose because they could not smell the confectionery or because they disliked sweet odours.

The researchers found a correlation between weight loss and the frequency of use of the odour inhaler and concluded that it is possible that smells can help sustain weight loss over a period of six months, when used with diet and exercise.

Dr Hirsch believes the effect arises because odours suppress hunger pangs or perhaps because they "break the Pavlovian conditioned response. You learn that the food smell does not necessarily mean food".

Dr Hirsch is now carrying out a one-year follow-up study of 12,000 people to extend the smells under investigation to cranberry, barbecued meat and cola, and to check if the weight loss can be sustained.

5. Therapies for obesity

Reasons for undergoing treatment to deal with obesity may include: the obesity itself, high blood pressure, heart and arterial disease, diabetes mellitus, joint problems, back pain, impending surgery or psychological problems.

Study activity 5

Collect information about various diets from magazines and have a group discussion about one of them. Be sure to discuss the following aspects:
- What is the composition of the diet?
- Can the diet be maintained for any length of time?
- Does the diet seem to be a suitable therapy for obesity?

Finding a therapy for obesity is not easy. A large number of the adults who start weight loss therapy do lose some weight but, after a while, many of them gain it again. Establishing new eating habits can be particularly useful, but it is also quite difficult, and the help of a dietitian is often required. Amongst the many treatments available for adiposity, the following general methods can be identified.

a. Weight-reducing diets

A balanced, low energy diet without special slimming products, herb teas, or miracle pills seems to be preferred. Diets which guarantee thinness, like the grapefruit diet and the bread lovers' diet are unbalanced and may even be harmful to the body over a long period of time. In addition, their results are usually only short-term because they do not improve eating behaviour and at the end of the diet most people relapse into their former eating habits and regain the weight quite quickly.

Special slimming products should only be used where there is serious obesity and even then only under medical supervision. As well as the disadvantage that they do not bring about change in eating habits, these products tend to be expensive.

b. Behaviour modification

This method is based on people coming to terms with their inappropriate eating behaviours, and is particularly suitable in cases of slight or moderate obesity. It is based on the assumption that being overweight is caused by 'wrong' eating behaviour, such as:
- eating because of boredom;
- eating food just because it is available;
- an inability to say 'no' when food is offered;
- missing meals;
- eating fast and chewing quickly;
- eating while you are standing, walking or watching television;
- always having two helpings;
- always having a snack at a particular time, such as when you come home from school or work;
- eating just before going to bed or late in the evening.

The ultimate goal of this method is to induce a permanent change in eating behaviour. One important feature of it is the 'dietary record', in which you note what, where and when you ate, who you were with and the mood you were in at the time. This encourages an awareness of eating behaviour, so that new habits and practices can be learned step by step.

c. Physical exercise

When combined with a low energy diet and behaviour modification, physical exercise offers some important advantages. It uses up energy and increases the metabolic rate. For example:
- the amount of energy provided by one slice of bread with cheese and one glass of semi-skimmed milk is equal to the amount of energy required for a one-hour walk;
- a soft drink (200 ml) provides enough energy for a 20-minute bike ride.

d. Slimming products

These include products such as medicines and appetite-depressants, massage creams for specific areas of fat in the body, herbal tea, enzyme pills or diuretic pills. These products are based largely on the power of suggestion in that if weight loss is expected, it tends to occur. Medicines which depress the appetite can cause undesirable side-effects, such as drowsiness or insomnia, irritability, and depression.

6. The low energy or weight-reducing diet

The most common method of treatment for obesity is the low energy or weight-reduction diet. This is directed chiefly at the basic cause of obesity (more energy is being consumed than the body is using) because the emphasis is on reducing the energy intake from food. However, attention will also have to be paid to the psychosocial factors underlying the obesity.

a. Goals and principles of the low energy diet
There are two goals in the low energy diet: it aims to improve eating behaviour and to achieve an attainable target weight. There are some important principles which should be followed if the low energy diet is to be successful. Some of these are listed below:
- The subject must be motivated to lose weight. It is important to be properly informed about the connection between obesity and other possible conditions. Often it is a doctor or a spouse who wants the subject to lose weight, while the individual in question does not feel any need to do so;
- The diet should help to improve eating behaviour, and ensure that the subject does not revert to former eating patterns. Support from family, friends, health care workers and others in close contact with the subject, will be particularly valuable;
- The aim is a healthy diet with less energy and the energy content can be reduced by decreasing the quantity of fats, carbohydrates and alcohol in the diet;
- Feelings of hunger can be partially counteracted by a generous intake of

products rich in dietary fibre, such as raw vegetables for snacks, or large portions of vegetables with meals. Eating more dietary fibre also helps to prevent constipation, which can occur as a result of a low energy diet. A large glass of water before every meal can reduce hunger pangs, and eating at regular times can also prevent feelings of hunger. It is recommended that everyone should eat three main meals per day, with small snacks between each meal. It is better to eat a little and often rather than sitting down to regular large meals.
- Food should be eaten slowly and chewed well to aid digestion and to increase awareness of what is being eaten;
- The diet should be tasty and varied, and adapted to the needs and preferences of the subject. This will make it much easier to adhere to the diet;
- The subject should not weigh him or herself more than once a week and this should be done first thing in the morning.

Study activity 6
a. If you wish to lose weight, there are two ways of doing it: lose as much weight as you can in the shortest possible time, or lose weight gradually over a longer period. Which do you think is the best method? Explain your answer.
b. Give five recommendations for maintaining the proper body weight.

b. Foodstuffs to avoid in a low energy diet
The low energy diet should be, essentially, a healthy diet. Food which provides a lot of energy should be avoided. These are foods which are rich in fat, sugar or alcohol, such as:
- full fat cheese, fatty meat products like salami, sausages, pies, sausage rolls and sandwich fillings;
- full fat milk, full fat yoghurt, readymade puddings;
- concentrated squash, soft drinks;

- thickened gravy, thickened soup;
- peanuts, crisps, nuts, savoury snacks;
- cakes, biscuits, pastries;
- all types of fatty meat;
- fatty fish (such as herring, salmon, mackerel, sardines);
- salad cream, mayonnaise;
- vegetables in a cream sauce;
- alcoholic beverages.

If the normal diet is reduced by 1,000 kcal or 4,200 kJ a day, then a weight loss of approximately 0.5 kg per week can be achieved.

Study activity 7

Make a list of foodstuffs which are suitable for a low energy diet, i.e. foods which contain little fat, sugar or alcohol.

Case study

Mrs Russell is a small 62-year-old woman and she is fairly overweight. She is 150 cm (5 ft) tall and weighs 73 kg (11^1/$_2$ stones). She was admitted to hospital for a knee operation, having suffered from painful and progressively weakening knees for a long time. The pain is aggravated by her weight and, in addition, she has fairly high blood pressure. She would like to lose weight if that would help to relieve her problems and, in consultation with a dietitian, the following low energy diet was devised. It has been adapted to her own eating habits as much as possible.

Low energy diet (4,200 kJ/1,000 kcal) for Mrs Russell
(Example of a day's menu)
Breakfast
- 1 slice of wholemeal bread (or 2 slices of crispbread) with low fat margarine and a little marmalade
- tea without sugar

Mid-morning snack
- coffee with a little milk but no sugar
- 1 digestive biscuit

Lunch
- thin soup
- 1 portion of lean meat or fish
- 2 small potatoes (boiled) with thin gravy
- generous portion of vegetables
- serving of salad
- 1 small portion of low fat yoghurt with pieces of fresh fruit.

Afternoon snack
- tea without sugar
- 1 glass of semi-skimmed milk or low fat yoghurt

Dinner
- 2 slices of wholemeal bread with low fat margarine and 1 slice of medium fat cheese or 1 slice of lean meat
- 1 boiled egg (twice a week) or baked beans or a small piece of grilled chicken
- 1 small bowl of low fat cottage cheese or quark with pieces of fresh fruit added.

Supper
- tea with a little milk but no sugar
- 1 portion of fresh fruit or 1 glass of fruit juice

To be taken whenever desired
   1 cup of low calorie soup, cups of tea, raw vegetables such as cucumber, carrots, tomatoes, courgettes, low calorie drinks and mineral water.

Study activity 8

a. Why is it important for Mrs Russell to lose weight?
b. For what other medical reasons can it be important to follow a low energy diet?
c. What goals should Mrs Russell's low energy diet be trying to attain?
d. Why are foodstuffs that are rich in dietary fibre suitable for a low energy diet? Give some examples of such foods.
e. Do you think the following would be suitable for Mrs Russell: sugar-free pastry, unsweetened fruit juice, white bread, cherries in syrup, cheddar cheese, soft drinks, low fat fruit yoghurt, tonic water, tomato juice? Explain your answer.

f. List three drinks which she can have without restriction. What snacks would you suggest for between meals?

g. Name three types of sandwich filling which are suitable for a low energy diet. What can you suggest in place of one slice of bread?

h. How often do you think Mrs Russell should weigh herself?

i. Her husband, who dislikes the idea of a diet, always brings her bars of chocolate. What action should be taken?

7. Summary

If we consume more energy than our body requires, we become overweight. Obesity beyond a certain level has obvious consequences for health. Treatment will be more successful if we know why people are eating more than they need to. Various physical, psychological and social factors can play a role.

Many people follow all sorts of diets which guarantee slimness, and they may do this for medical reasons or for fashion trends. The values of various slimming therapies were discussed. The low energy diet is the most common diet used in health care, and the aims and principles of this diet were explored in some detail. It is, however, very important in any weight loss programme for attention to be paid to the psychosocial factors which underlie the obesity problem.

Final test for module 3

Instructions

This section consists of 50 statements or sentences. Each one may be correct or incorrect. The answer required is either YES or NO.

In your assessment of whether one of the 50 items is correct or not, you should base your answers only on the circumstances and facts given.

The questions are arranged in groups, in the order that the related topics occurred in the text. After ensuring that all the questions have been answered, check the results of the test yourself using the answers at the back of the book.

1. In Britain there are more illnesses resulting from malnutrition than illnesses resulting from unbalanced diets with an excess of fats and sugars.
2. Risk factors for heart and arterial diseases include high blood pressure and a high cholesterol level.
3. The most fatty foodstuffs contain unsaturated fat.
4. Sunflower oil and diet margarine used instead of butter can help to lower the cholesterol level.
5. Vegetables, fruit, meat and wholemeal bread all contain a lot of dietary fibre.
6. Limiting fat consumption in the diet can help to prevent cancer.
7. A diet low in dietary fibre can give rise to constipation and haemorrhoids.
8. Diverticulosis is a disorder of the intestinal lining whereby sacs are formed. This is caused by too much dietary fibre.
9. You need several spoonfuls of bran in your daily diet.
10. Anorexia nervosa is particularly common among females aged between 14 and 25.
11. Bulimia nervosa does not occur among men.
12. People with anorexia nervosa may also have eating binges.
13. Bulimia nervosa is an eating disorder in which great quantities of food are consumed in a short period of time.
14. People suffering from bulimia nervosa always end their eating binges with vomiting or the use of laxatives.
15. Therapy for anorexia nervosa or bulimia nervosa can be made more effective if focused primarily on the psychosocial problems.
16. The following recommendation may be useful during therapy for anorexia or bulimia nervosa: 'If you are angry, get into a rage instead of trying to eat away your anger or convert it into not eating. Otherwise you only deny those feelings and you will not solve anything.'
17. Frozen products are best defrosted by running them under hot water.
18. Frozen vegetables should be defrosted before they are cooked.
19. The symptoms of food poisoning normally occur within eight hours and they usually consist of nausea and vomiting.
20. Most pathogenic bacteria and those which cause food to spoil are destroyed when heated above 60°C.

21. Frozen products are free from bacteria as long as they are stored properly.
22. Beer in an unopened bottle can be kept for an unlimited amount of time.
23. Removing the mould from a fruit preserve makes it safe to eat.
24. The proper temperature for a refrigerator is 10°C.
25. Dried figs and dates can 'go off' quickly.
26. It is best to keep leftover vegetables refrigerated in a tin.
27. Milk which is not stored in a dark place will lose its vitamins.
28. It is better not to reheat leftover spinach.
29. White bits in honey show that it is of inferior quality.
30. There is nothing wrong with refreezing frozen pastry which has already been defrosted.
31. The water from thawed meat can be used to prepare gravy.
32. Food which is contaminated with bacteria always smells or tastes worse than uncontaminated food.
33. Bacteria tend to live in foodstuffs rich in protein and water and not in dry, sweet, or salty food.
34. Frozen food should be defrosted in the refrigerator unless otherwise indicated on the packaging.
35. A preservative is an example of a contaminant.
36. Examples of vegetables rich in nitrate include celery and cabbage.
37. A toasted sandwich with burnt, black patches contains carcinogenic substances.
38. Diet margarine is a suitable item for a low energy diet.
39. In order to lose weight, it would be better to eat fresh fruit rather than fruit juice.
40. Acidic foods, like lemons, pickles and grapefruit, help to remove the fat from your body.
41. Potatoes make you fat.
42. Serious obesity increases the risk of high blood pressure, diabetes, joint problems and varicose veins.
43. A good way to lose weight is to shed as much weight as possible over the shortest possible period.
44. Reducing the energy intake in your diet involves limiting the consumption of fats, carbohydrates, water, and salt.
45. Fat around the stomach area is more harmful for your health than fat on the hips.
46. Tonic water and bitter lemon are soft drinks which contain only a little sugar.
47. You can often lose weight by simply avoiding snacks.
48. A good way to lose weight is to miss a meal.
49. Black coffee without sugar provides no energy.
50. Slimming creams for massaging into the body melt away the fat under the skin.

References and further reading

Agras W S (ed), (1987) *Management of Obesity, Bulimia and Anorexia Nervosa.* Pergamon Press, Oxford.

Committee on Medical Aspects of Food Policy (COMA), (1987) *Diet and Cardiovascular Disease.* HMSO, London.

Craddock D, (1987) *Obestiy and its Management.* Churchill Livingstone, Edinburgh.

DHSS, (1981) *Report on Avoiding Heart Attacks.* HMSO, London.

Frohlich E, (1990) *Preventative Aspects of Coronary Heart Disease.* FA Davis, Philadelphia.

Garrow J and Webster J, (1985) Quetelet's index as a measure of fatness. *International Journal of Obesity,* 9, 147-153.

Gilbert S, (1989) *Psychology of Dieting.* Routledge, London.

Lenfant C, (1990) The cholesterol facts. *American Association of Occupational Health Nurses Journal,* 38, (5), 209-210.

National Dairy Council and MORI, (1992) *Food and Health: What does Britian Think?* NDC, London.

National Food Survey Committee Annual Report, (1991) *Household Food Consumption and Expenditure.* HMSO, London.

Scotland's Health, (1993) *A Challenge to us All. The Scottish Diet. Report of a Working Party to the Chief Medical Officer for Scotland,* HMSO, Edinburgh.

Scott D, (1988) *Anorexia and Bulimia Nervosa: Practical Approaches.* Croom Helm, London.

Smith A and Jacobson B, (1988) *The Nation's Health - A Strategy for the 1990s.* Oxford University Press, Oxford.

Module 4

OTHER INFLUENCES ON THE DIET

Introduction Module 4

In the previous chapters we have seen that we should eat less food in general, and certainly less fat, sugar and salt. Some people, however, set themselves far more stringent targets, consciously choosing a diet which differs from our normal eating habits. This is known as an 'alternative diet', and health care workers are often confronted with patients who have chosen to adopt such a diet. Young people in particular may have alternative eating habits. There are, of course, many different forms of alternative diet, but in this module we will only discuss the most popular ones.

The module then discusses the eating habits of some ethnic minority groups, particularly those of the Asian, Afro-Caribbean, Jewish, and Chinese communities. Their diets cannot be described as alternative because their choices of food and modes of preparation are traditional to their specific cultures.

Alternative nutrition

1

1. Introduction

Alternative nutrition has been gaining stature in the past few years among both consumers and producers and this is evident in the High Street of any British town with the notable increase in the number of organic food shops, health food shops and the like. The term 'health food' is somewhat unfortunate because it implies something which is necessary for, and which improves health. There is really no such thing as a health food, just a health food industry which is, in fact, worth £220 million per annum.

The people who follow an alternative diet may also demonstrate an increased awareness of some aspects of life on which, formerly, little importance was placed. For instance, they reflect an increased concern for living things and the environment and there is often a desire to live in greater harmony with nature. In general, the various types of alternative nutrition which are dealt with in this chapter can be considered healthy, as long as appropriate choices are made.

Learning outcomes

After studying this chapter the student should be able to:
– explain what is meant by an alternative diet;
– list six reasons for following an alternative diet;
– explain the difference between a vegetarian and a vegan;
– describe how to formulate a healthy diet without meat;
– give short descriptions of organic, macrobiotic and anthroposophic diets;
– explain the principles of organic agricultural methods.

2. Alternative nutrition

In general, we can say that an alternative diet is a dietary pattern which is different from the typical diet of that society. In alternative diets, meals are compiled according to different principles, some of which may include the partial or complete rejection of animal products. In this chapter we will discuss the following alternative diets:
– the organic food diet
– the macrobiotic diet
– the anthroposophic diet.

Study activity 1

a. Do you, personally, sometimes have a day without meat? Why, or why not?

b. What reasons can you think of why people follow a meat-free diet?

c. Refer to Figure 4.1.1. Discuss the pros and cons of farming animals like this in Britain.

a. Reasons for following an alternative diet
People follow alternative diets for a variety of reasons: health concerns, fear of additives, influence of media, 'quick' health, improved appearance, perceived cure for illnesses. Another of the reasons for following an alternative dietary pattern is religious belief, as in the following example.

Case study

The Seventh Day Adventists, an American religious group, attach a great deal of value to living a healthy life. They do not smoke nor drink alcohol, and they live according to the Laws of Moses. Their church also gives advice about choice of foods and eating behaviour. The most important guidelines are:

- follow a vegetarian diet
- take as much unprocessed food as possible, such as wholemeal bread, fresh vegetables, fruit and brown rice
- avoid spices and drinks containing caffeine, or take them only in moderation.

Figure 4.1.1
© Daily Telegraph 13/10/93

RSPCA issues care code as ostrich farming takes off

by Robert Bedlow

OSTRICH farming in Britain is causing such "great concern" to the RSPCA that the society issued guidelines yesterday on how to care for the flightless creatures.

With eggs costing up to £1,000 each, chicks worth more than £2,000, and adult breeding birds fetching between £20,000 and £30,000, interest in *Struthio camaelus*, the world's largest living bird, has soared.

Since ostrich eggs began to be imported to Britain from Namibia three years ago, the number of birds in the country has risen to 300, the majority being chicks and juveniles raised on about 20 farms.

Mr Mark Ranson, RSPCA scientific officer, said:

"While we're concerned that a new species is being farmed in this country, we are doing all we can to make sure ostriches escape the kind of abuse that has gone on in other livestock production areas."

The ostrich is found mainly in Africa, but can be kept outdoors in Britain in all but the worst weathers, when shelter must be provided.

They are gregarious birds and should never be kept on their own. They can reach speeds of 40mph and should have at least a quarter of an acre to roam. No more than 15 should be allowed in a one-acre paddock.

Feathers should never be pulled from a living bird and all farms must have their own slaughterhouse – sending ostriches to an abattoir would cause distress, the guidelines say.

Owners are also reminded that the bird, which can deliver a kick as bruising as a Nigel Benn punch, has to be registered under the 1976 Dangerous Wild Animals Act.

The birds – an adult male 8ft tall, weighs about 340lb, females slightly smaller and lighter – are used mainly for breeding, but some are killed for their meat and the hide, which produces a soft, fine-grained leather.

Mr Francis Ayres, and his wife Linda, who have an ostrich farm near Banbury, Oxon, have invested £40,000 in an effort to persuade consumers that the meat is safe and healthy. "It has a venison-like flavour," said Mr Ayres,

Research has shown that, compared with the average American, cancer occurs less often amongst Seventh Day Adventists. In addition, they suffer from less heart and arterial disease. Reasons for this include their alternative dietary pattern, regular physical exercise, the avoidance of stress and also their non-smoking lifestyle.

Maintaining health is itself a popular motive for following an alternative diet and, where this is the case, people often attach a great deal of value to eating food which has undergone as little industrial processing as possible (such as being free from chemical additives) and which has been produced without artificial fertilisers or pesticides. Some people also choose an alternative diet because of their concern for the environment. They may believe that the production and distribution of food should not have such a high cost environmentally, and their goal is to live more harmoniously with nature. A number of people follow alternative diets as part of a course of alternative medical treatment such as homeopathy, philosophical medicine or natural medicine.

b. The vegetarian diet

A vegetarian diet does not contain any food which has been obtained by the killing of animals, and there are two basic vegetarian groups: vegans (or strict vegetarians) who eat no animal products whatsoever, and avoid milk, other dairy products and eggs; and vegetarians (or lacto-ovo-vegetarians) who do not eat meat or fish, but they will eat eggs, milk, and other dairy products.

Vegetarian products are usually clearly marked and some manufacturers use their own symbol which identifies the product as vegetarian. However, companies can approach the Vegetarian Society, who can approve ingredients as suitable for vegetarians, and allow such companies to use the V.S. logo (see Figure 4.1.2).

Figure 4.1.2
Approved by the Vegetarian Society

People eat meat for many reasons such as the taste, the status associated with it, or the high protein content for instance. There are just as many reasons why someone might choose *not* to eat meat, one of the main ones being a moral objection to the killing of animals. In addition, however, many people avoid meat because of its high cost, or because they simply do not like the taste.

Examples of foods usually avoided by vegetarians include: meat, fish, game, poultry, shellfish, ordinary margarine, frying fats containing fat from animal sources, gelatine (derived from bones), meat stock cubes and ready-made soups and sauces from tins or packets. In addition, a vegan will not take milk, dairy products, eggs, honey or any products containing these.

Figure 4.1.3
Battery chickens

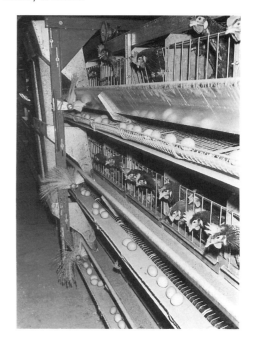

Figure 4.1.4
Freedom Food, July 1994

Freedom Food Ltd has been set up by the RSPCA as a wholly-owned subsidiary to improve farm animal welfare standards.
Farmers, hauliers and abattoirs will be inspected by specialist Freedom Food assessors. RSPCA technical and scientific staff will also be making spot checks.
Everyone meeting these standards will be able to use the Freedom Food Trademark.

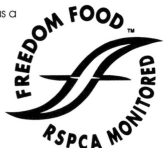

Figure 4.1.5
The RSPCA Farm Animal Welfare Standards for Freedom Food, July 1994

The RSPCA Farm Animal Welfare Standards for Freedom Food

A Summary

The RSPCA has produced welfare standards for farm animals as a pro-active approach to provide producers, hauliers, abattoirs and processors with guidance of how best to look after their stock – and thereby enable them to join the Freedom Food scheme.

Freedom Food is based upon the Five Freedoms, which describe the ideal welfare conditions for animals throughout their lives.

The Five Freedoms are:
- Freedom from hunger and thirst
  - by ready access to fresh water and a diet to maintain full health and vigour
- Freedom from discomfort
  - by providing an appropriate environment including shelter and a comfortable resting area
- Freedom from pain, injury or disease
  - by prevention or rapid diagnosis and treatment
- Freedom to express normal behaviour
  - by producing sufficient space, proper facilities and company of the animal's own kind
- Freedom from fear and distress
  - by ensuring conditions and care which avoid mental suffering

These freedoms will be better provided for if those who have care of livestock practise

The Five Obligations:
- Caring and responsible planning and management
- Skilled, knowledgeable and conscientious stockmanship
- Appropriate environmental design
- Considerate handling and transport
- Humane slaughter

c. Free range produce

There is also a large number of people who are worried about the quality of factory-farmed meat, because it can contain residues of veterinary medication and growth hormones. Factory-farming is also often condemned because of the conditions in which the animals live. For example, a battery chicken lives its entire life in an area 20cm square (Figure 4.1.3). Rabbits are kept in an even smaller area, and are killed when they are 12 weeks old. In addition, current factory farming practices can be harmful to the environment because of the excessive production of manure.

Consequently some people will only eat the meat or produce of animals which they know have had a more humane life, and this is often sold under the description 'free range' meat or eggs. In the United Kingdom the Ministry of Agriculture, Fisheries and Food monitors free range eggs to ensure that they comply with all the rules and codes of practice as laid down by the European Union relating to the production, processing, and trading of free range eggs.

Study activity 2

a. Do you have any strong views on free range meat and eggs?
b. What do you think about the RSPCA initiative outlined above?

d. How can you plan a balanced diet without meat?

Meat is rich in protein, iron and B vitamins. Consequently, if meat is not included in the diet it is important to pay particular attention to these nutrients (Figure 4.1.6).

We usually obtain more than enough protein from sources other than meat. It is also found in milk and other dairy products, pulses, eggs, cereals, bread, nuts and, to a lesser extent, potatoes; this makes it almost impossible for anyone with a varied and balanced diet to suffer from a protein deficiency.

Figure 4.1.6
Some substitutes for meat

	Protein (g)	Iron (mg)
75g cheese	17	0.3
2 eggs	13	2.0
100 pulses (40g dried)	8	2.4
150g cooked cereal (50g dried)	4	2.5
200g soya bean curd	15	2.4
80g nuts	14	2.4
100g peanut butter	23	2.1
For comparison:		
100g meat	18	2.5

Meat is also an important source of iron. It is therefore important for people who do not eat meat to make sure that they do eat foodstuffs containing a lot of iron. Examples of such foodstuffs include: wholemeal products (wholemeal bread, dark rye bread, brown rice, wholewheat macaroni, wholewheat spaghetti, muesli and porridge), pulses, vegetables, eggs, and nuts. The B vitamins that are found in meat are also found in milk, wholemeal cereals, pulses, eggs, and vegetables. Vegans seldom suffer from a vitamin B deficiency. However, women who are pregnant or breast-feeding need extra B vitamins, so their diet may have to be supplemented with a vitamin B_{12} preparation.

Example of a vegetarian bread-based meal
–   wholemeal bread, nut bread
     with vegetable margarine
     or
     with cheese, peanut butter, hummus
     or jam
–   raw vegetables
–   yoghurt with pieces of pear
–   tea

Examples of a vegetarian hot meal
– baked banana
– brown rice with peanut sauce
– tomato and cucumber salad
– yoghurt with pieces of apple and raisins
    or
– bubble and squeak, an economical dish made by frying a left-over mixture of cooked cabbage and potatoes
– chicory salad
– yoghurt with strawberries

Examples of a hot meal for vegans
– stuffed pepper (with rice, lentils, mushrooms)
– baked potatoes
– leeks
– oranges
    or
– casserole with brown beans
– brown rice and vegetables
– salad with carrots, apple and walnuts

Study activity 3

Plan a hot meal for a vegetarian and another for a vegan.

3. The organic food diet

The basic principle behind the organic food diet is that man and his environment are dependent on each other. The term 'organic food' is a fairly ambiguous term. However, organic food should meet a set standard such as that set by the Soil Association. Before produce can carry the Association's symbol, the land it was grown on must have been free from chemical fertilisers for 2 years or more. The organic food diet is, therefore, not only concerned with assuring the health and well-being of the individual, but also with maintaining a healthy environment.

The organic food diet differs from the average diet in that enormous value is attached to those agricultural practices that place as small a burden as possible on nature. For example, no chemical pesticides or artificial fertiliser should be used. Produce conforming to these standards is described as 'organically grown', and in general it contains less nitrate than produce grown using artificial fertiliser. This is of benefit to the consumer, as nitrate can be concentrated in the body into nitrosamines which have demonstrated

Figure 4.1.7
The Soil Association

carcinogenic effects in laboratory animals. The disadvantages of a diet too high in nitrate were discussed in detail in Module 3, Chapter 3.

Organic food is also normally processed in an environmentally friendly way, and it should undergo as little industrial processing as possible because this causes loss of vitamins, minerals and dietary fibre, as has happened in highly processed foods such as white bread, wheat flour, cornflour and white rice. People who are concerned about ecology are also often critical of the way additives are used in food since, by improving the appearance of a product they give the consumer a false impression.

A lot of energy can be saved by buying food that is grown locally and which is seasonal, such as Brussels sprouts or leeks in the winter, and the many varieties of fruits and vegetables which are available in the summer. In order to grow tomatoes in winter much energy is needed to heat greenhouses, and produce imported from abroad requires a lot of fuel for transport. For environmental reasons, many people also prefer food to have the least possible packaging, and any packaging necessary should be either biodegradable (such as paper bags) or else reusable.

The Soil Association regulates the production of organic foods, and no produce may be labelled 'organic' without their approval.

Study activity 4

a. What disadvantages might there be in following a diet rich in organic foods?
b. Plan a full meat-containing meal and a similar organic one. Compare the advantages and disadvantages of each.

4. Macrobiotics

Macrobiotics is a philosophy based on prolonging life and improving its quality, and diet is an important part of its practices. The ideal is that every person should live in individual harmony with nature. The ancient Chinese concepts of Yin and Yang (Figure 4.1.8) which are held to be the basis of all things and therefore found in all things, offer a useful way of looking at balance in the diet (Figure 4.1.9).

Figure 4.1.9
Yin and Yang balance

Yin represents	Yang represents
growing	shrinking
cold	hot
passive	active
feminine	masculine
wet	dry
fast	slow
fruit	cheese
butter	meat
milk	fish
vegetables	eggs

Figure 4.1.8
Yin and Yang symbol

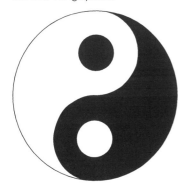

Yin and Yang are complementary, opposing forces like day and night, man and woman, hard and soft, fat and thin, fire and water, solid and fluid. Taken together, each pair forms a unified whole, but one cannot exist without the other. For health and harmony, the two opposing forces must be in balance, and illness occurs when there is an imbalance between them.

This Yin-Yang division is also used to classify foodstuffs. With a few exceptions, vegetables have more Yin than do animal foods; fruit, green vegetables and sweet-and-sour tasting products are particularly associated with Yin, while meat, fish, salt, and bitter foods are associated with Yang. The main components of the diet should be cereals, pulses or seeds, carrots, or green vegetables and products like miso and tofu (which are made from soya beans and sea salt); animal products like honey, dairy produce, fish and meat should only be eaten in very moderate quantities.

Until recently, the emphasis of macrobiotics was on the healing effects of a diet which consisted entirely of cereals, and such a diet had to be implemented over a long period of time to be effective. However, in practice, such diets have resulted in serious nutritional deficiencies and in dehydration. Today, such a diet is almost never used for healing and when it is, it would only be over short periods. Nevertheless, a person following the guidelines for a macrobiotic diet can satisfy all their nutritional requirements. Furthermore, such a diet contains little sugar, fat, or salt and only a moderate amount of protein, and consequently it can contribute to the prevention of diseases related to the excesses of the Western diet.

5. Anthroposophy

Anthroposophy is a philosophy developed by Rudolf Steiner (1861-1925) and within it the choice of food is based on far more than the concept of nutrition. The whole image of the person must be taken into account when selecting a diet, and this image consists of three parts: the body, the soul and the spirit (these may also be called the will, the feeling and the thinking). Each of these parts corresponds to a particular part of a plant. Figure 4.1.10 shows which sections of the plant correspond to the parts making up a person's whole image.

Figure 4.1.10
The anthroposophical correlation between plants and the person

Part of plant	Body	Mind
root and tuber	nerves, senses	thinking
leaf and stem	heart, lungs	feeling
fruit, seed, flower	metabolism, limbs	will

According to Figure 4.1.10, a diet of root vegetables will improve the powers of the mind, while a diet with a lot of green vegetables will benefit breathing and blood circulation. For anthroposophists, meals often consist of a carefully varied composition of different plant parts, including roots or tubers, leaves, flowers, fruit, and seeds.

6. Are alternative diets healthy?

Compared to the average diet, a vegetarian, organic, macrobiotic, or anthroposophic diet usually contains less energy, less saturated fat, less salt and sugar, and more starch and dietary fibre. Such diets can help to prevent the illnesses associated with the current Western diet which were discussed in Module 3, Chapter 1. In addition, alternative diets often contain fewer of the harmful substances like alcohol and caffeine, and fewer pesticides, additives, pollutants, and other potentially harmful substances. However, vegetarian diets may be low in iron and vegan diets low in calcium. The level of fluid intake requires particular attention in children, the elderly, and the ill, and in these groups the macrobiotic guideline to 'drink only when thirsty' may lead to kidney dysfunction and symptoms of dehydration. In general, therefore, alternative dietary patterns can be considered healthy, but there is a risk if they are not followed sensibly.

Study activity 5

Consider Figure 4.1.11. Discuss in your group the conclusions which might be drawn from the article.

7. Summary

Many people, particularly the young, choose a dietary pattern which differs from the norm or food from 'alternative' sources. This means that at some point health care workers are likely to have to deal with such diets. The most common alternative diets are the vegetarian diet, the organic food diet, the macrobiotic diet, and the anthroposophic diet. One notable common factor is the partial or total exclusion of animal products.

The reasons for following such diets may include concern for health, concern for the environment, opposition to factory-farming, religious conviction, or a certain philosophy of life. Such diets generally have an adequate nutritional composition provided that appropriate choices of food are made within the constraints of each diet. They also help to prevent many of the diseases associated with the excesses of our Western diet, and they usually contain fewer harmful substances. In addition, they are generally better for the environment. One important disadvantage for many people, however, is the high cost of much of this alternative produce.

Figure 4.1.11
© The Guardian 24/6/94

Vegetarian diet reduces risk of early death, study concludes

Chris Mihill, Medical Correspondent

VEGETARIANS are nearly 40 per cent less likely to die of cancer and 30 per cent less likely to die of heart disease than meat eaters, according to a study published today in the British Medical Journal.

Although there have been previous reports that a vegetarian diet is more healthy, questions about death rates have been confused because other aspects of lifestyle could be contributing. The new research has excluded factors such as smoking, obesity and socio-economic status and still concludes vegetarians are less prone to early death.

Stephen Connor, campaign director for the Vegetarian Society, said last night: "Study after study has shown that a vegetarian diet is healthier ... There is only one conclusion: the meat industry kills more than just animals. For your health's sake, go veggie."

Amanda Weir, a nutritionist with the Meat and Livestock Commission, said: "The authors of the study say themselves there is no evidence that people should give up meat."

The study, one of the largest yet attempted, followed 6,115 vegetarians over a 12-year period and compared their death rates with those of 5,015 meat eaters. Overall, there was a 20 per cent less chance of death from all causes over the 12 years for the vegetarians. Vegetarians had a 39 per cent lower risk of death from cancer, and 29 per cent lower risk of death from heart disease.

The researchers – Barbara Thorogood, Klim McPherson and Jim Mann, of the London School of Hygiene and Tropical Medicine, and Paul Appleby, of Oxford University – point out that apart from a high vegetable and fruit intake, vegetarians have a diet rich in cereals, pulses and nuts, eat less saturated fat and more carbohydrate and dietary fibre, and have a higher intake of antioxidant vitamins,

There has been much interest amongst cancer specialists and heart disease researchers into the protective effects of a vegetarian-style or Mediterranean-type diet. The study has been funded by the Cancer Research Campaign and the Imperial Cancer Research Fund. The researchers say that people should not abandon meat entirely, but should eat more fruit and vegetables.

Figure 4.1.12
Vegetarian food labels

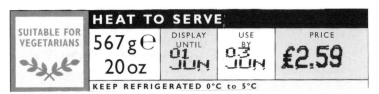

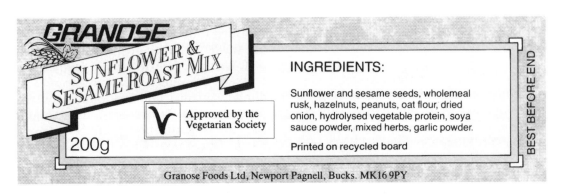

INGREDIENTS:

Sunflower and sesame seeds, wholemeal rusk, hazelnuts, peanuts, oat flour, dried onion, hydrolysed vegetable protein, soya sauce powder, mixed herbs, garlic powder.

Printed on recycled board

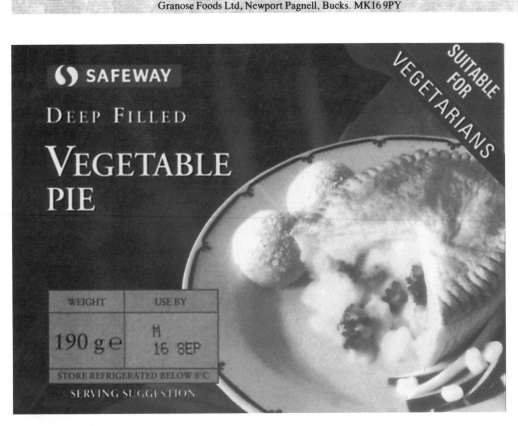

Diet, religion, and ethnic communities

1. Introduction

Britain is regarded as a multinational and multicultural society. The 1991 census shows that 6% of the population in England and Wales are of ethnic minority origin, and that the total number of black and ethnic minority population is likely to double over the next 40 to 50 years. People from different backgrounds often enjoy diets which correspond to their traditions, religion, or both. It is, therefore, very useful to have a particular knowledge of the lifestyles and dietary habits of the different ethnic groups in our society in order to help us to communicate better with the patients we meet.

Learning outcomes

After studying this chapter students should be able to:
– understand what factors must be taken into consideration when planning diets for clients from ethnic minorities during a stay in a hospital or nursing home.

2. The diets of ethnic minority groups

Many people from different ethnic or religious groups try to retain the eating habits of their particular religion or culture, and food from a wide variety of cultures can often be found in markets and specialist shops, particularly in the larger cities in Britain. Changes in eating habits do occur over time as societies influence each other, but the traditional methods for preparing their food are still used and enjoyed. Certainly, Western food has been considerably enhanced by the addition of Asian, Italian, Chinese, Caribbean and other types of cookery.

3. The Islamic or Muslim diet

Most of the Muslims in Britain originated from Pakistan, Bangladesh, and other Asian and Middle Eastern countries. In Islamic communities, religion has a considerable influence on the choice of food and the mode of preparation. Food has a very important social function and cooking and eating are esteemed social activities.

The Koran, the holy book of Islam, contains many rules and regulations regarding food. It forbids Muslims to eat pork, and the meat of other animals such as cows, sheep, or chickens may only be eaten if all the blood is drained from the carcass when the animal is killed. Muslims, therefore, prefer to buy their meat from an Islamic butcher because they can then be sure that the rules of the Koran have been observed. The Koran prohibits the use of alcohol, states that hands must be washed before eating (it is their custom to eat with their hands and usually from a communal plate, unless there is illness in the family), and that the person eating should only consume two-thirds of the quantity actually desired.

One of the major Muslim events is Ramadan, the month of fasting. During Ramadan, Muslims do not eat, drink, or take medication between sunrise and sunset. However, children under 12 and the chronically ill may be exempt from participating in the fasting. Others suffering from illness, together with women who are pregnant or breast-feeding, may postpone their period of fasting.

Everyday diet
Muslims are accustomed to eating one cold meal and two hot meals each day. They generally spend a lot of time preparing their meals, buying fresh produce and very few pre-prepared products. Bread is eaten with every hot meal and, in fact, for a Muslim a meal would be incomplete without bread.

The typical diet is similar to the Hindu diet (see below) and traditionally, meals consist mainly of peas, beans, lentils and other pulses with meat, chicken and fish. Dishes are accompanied with a variety of foodstuffs including rice, chapatis, paratha or naan bread, bhaji (chopped vegetables mixed in a spicy batter and deep fried), pakora (similar to bhaji), spinach, okra, tomato, potato, sweet potato, aubergine, cauliflower, cabbage, onion, and other vegetables. The food is normally highly spiced with ingredients such as coriander, turmeric, ginger, garlic, garam masala, chillies, cardamom seeds and cumin seeds. Natural yoghurt, chutneys and pickles are often home-made and accompany meals along with salads. After meals fresh fruit is served and very sweet cakes and sweetmeats, either home-made or from good Asian grocers.

4. The Hindu diet

Most of the Hindus in Britain originated in India. The most significant differences between the Hindu and Muslim diets are that orthodox Hindus are vegetarian while Muslims may eat meat (except pork) as long as the animal is ritually slaughtered. For Hindus, the cow is a sacred animal and so beef or veal in the diet are strictly forbidden. When Hindus eat meat, it is usually mutton, goat, chicken, and occasionally pork, and most of them will not eat fish. Those who observe the religion strictly are vegetarian, and will not eat eggs because they are a source of life, although they are allowed to eat dairy products. Fasting is an important element in Hindu religious practice, with a number of fasting days (from sunrise to sunset) in each month. On these days only pure foods are eaten outwith the daylight hours, such as fruit, yoghurt, or only fluids. Individuals can decide for themselves when it is an appropriate time to fast, and the position of the stars is often used as a guide, with an individual's own birth-star determining the starting point. Fasting is also part of the preparation for religious festivals.

Everyday diet
Hindus usually eat three meals a day and it is not customary for the whole family to eat together at set times. The first meal is usually eaten late in the morning, between 10 a.m. and 12 noon. Food is eaten either with the fingers of the right hand or with a spoon or fork.

Breakfast This may consist of white bread with butter or margarine, together with a choice of cheese, peanut butter, or jam.

Lunch This will be similar to breakfast.

Dinner Dinner often consists of rice with vegetables, pulses such as lentils, peas, or beans, and meat such as chicken, salted meat or dried salted fish. Potatoes and other root vegetables, such as sweet potatoes, cassava, and yams, often form part of a hot meal, as do cooked or fried bananas or plantains. Roti is a thin pancake that can be filled with vegetables, potatoes, and meat. The food must not have been in contact with beef or veal so meat stock cubes or powders are never used. Vegetables and meat are often fried in oil with the wide range of herbs and spices which was mentioned above.

Snacks between meals These may consist of fruit, a hard-boiled egg, samosas, biscuits or chocolate. Drinks will often be water or home-made lemonade, tea, coffee, or milk.

Figure 4.2.1
Norms and values are different in every culture

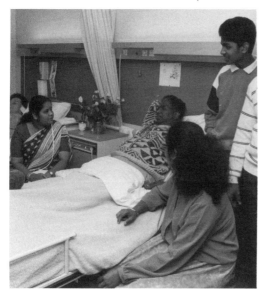

Figure 4.2.2

Vegetable Pilau

Ingredients:
2 cups rice washed and drained
3 cups water
1/2 cup undiluted evaporated milk mixed with 2 tsp lime juice to curdle it
1 tbsp ground sweet almonds
2 clusters coriander leaves
3 tbsp butter or margarine or a mixture of the two or ghee
2 tbsp finely diced onion
2 tbsp finely shredded ginger
4 cloves garlic, finely sliced
1 tbsp powdered turmeric mixed with 1/4 cup water

Vegetables –
2 cups cauliflower, cut into 3cm (1¹/₄ in) pieces, taking care to keep some of the stalk
1 large carrot, peeled, halved lengthwise and coarsely sliced
3/4 cup frozen green peas or green beans, cut into 2.5cm (1in) lengths

Method
First prepare the vegetable mixture to be added to the pilau,

Heat 1 tbsp butter (from amount specified) in saucepan. Add 2 tsp of the diced onion and a little of the shredded ginger and sliced garlic. When slightly brown, add all the vegetables, a little salt and 1/2 cup water, cover pan and cook on medium heat for about 10 minutes, taking care the vegetables do not burn. Remove the vegetables to a dish.

Now cook the rice.

In the same deep saucepan, heat the rest of the butter and fry the rest of the diced onion, the ginger and garlic till golden brown. Add the rice, stir and fry for a few minutes before adding salt and 3 cups of water. Cover pan and simmer on medium heat till water is absorbed by the rice. Mix the curdled milk and ground almonds to a smooth paste, adding a little water if too thick, and stir this gently into the rice. Put on top of the rice all the cooked vegetables and the 2 clusters of coriander leaves. Cover pan and simmer on very low heat till time to serve, gently mixing the vegetables and turmeric paste with the rice before spreading rice on platter.

Study activity

A 72-year-old Muslim woman has been in hospital for a month. She was admitted to the orthopaedic ward for assessment after breaking her hip, and since her admission she has eaten very little. She hardly speaks any English, but she has been able to let people know that she does not like the food she has been served. She is finding it very difficult to adapt to the situation, but when her family come to visit her mood changes and she is able to laugh again.

a. List three dietary factors that you would take into account in this situation.

b. Which of the following would the woman be able to eat?
Cheese made from sheep's milk, olives, mutton, couscous, chicken, beef, pork, sausage, bacon, ham, yoghurt, mint tea, fried banana, rice, salad oil, olive oil, chillies, wine.

c. If the woman in the example was a Hindu, what would the three important dietary factors be?

d. Which of the items listed above would a Hindu woman be able to eat?

e. In Islamic society, people are not normally *invited* to dinner. Food is always served when visitors come and everyone eats together. It is automatically assumed that the visitor will stay for dinner. What do you think of this custom?

5. The Jewish diet

There has been a Jewish community in Britain for centuries, and health care workers who deal with Jewish patients should be aware of the dietary rules and customs which are part of the Jewish religion whether or not they are strictly adhered to by the individual. There are only a few thousand Jews in Britain who live according to traditional, orthodox doctrine.

Traditional Jewish food does not seem to differ significantly from ordinary British food, but the Jewish religion has rules about the modes of food preparation, which makes the cooking and serving of food more involved. Jews believe that the laws governing food preparation are made by God, and are specifically meant to keep humans pure and holy through self-control and moderation. These laws are known as kashrut, and are as follows:

– Meat must not be purchased from an ordinary butcher. Animals must be killed in a special manner, the blood from the meat being drained off, and the meat soaked and salted before preparation;

– Pork is forbidden but beef, mutton, goat, and chicken are allowed;

– Fish with fins and scales can be eaten; smooth fish like eel cannot; shellfish and crustaceans are also considered unclean and must not be eaten;

– Dairy and meat products may not be eaten at the same sitting. This separation of meat and dairy products has the most significant influence on Jewish daily life. If meat is eaten, then dairy products such as milk, yoghurt, butter, cheese or cream cannot be eaten until at least one hour later. On the other hand, meat may be eaten *after* a dairy product, but only if the mouth has been cleansed and a piece of bread or fruit has been eaten first. In practice, an orthodox Jew will have certain plates, cutlery, kitchenware, and tablecloths reserved for use with meat products and others reserved for use with dairy products. Kitchenware and tableware are similarly washed separately and then stored in separate cupboards;

– Wine made by non-Jews is forbidden.

Food that has been prepared according to these laws is called *kosher* (clean). Every year, a list of approved foods, known as the *kashrut list*, is published in the Jewish Almanac. This list is compiled under rabbinical supervision. Examples of typical foodstuffs are Wiener schnitzel (veal), chicken soup, potatoes, shredded carrot, stewed fruit, minestrone soup, beef stew, cauliflower, lettuce, cucumber.

In the Jewish religion, there are a large number of holidays to which specific rules regarding diet are attached, i.e. during Pesach (the Jewish Easter), no leavened bread may be eaten nor even kept in the house. On these days, *matzos* – thin crackers made of wheat flour and water – are eaten instead of bread. The Jewish Sabbath starts on Friday night when it gets dark and lasts for 24 hours, during which time no fire may be lit. This means that soups or stews are prepared beforehand and placed in the oven before the Sabbath begins.

6. The Afro-Caribbean diet

Afro-Caribbeans are people of African descent who come from the Caribbean Islands. Eating practices and customs may differ between the islands, as would customs from different parts of Asia.

Generally, a number of basic ingredients are common in the diets of all Afro-Caribbean people. Cereals include corn, rice, oats, and wheat, with indigenous breads being a feature of their diet. Starchy fruits including green bananas, plantain, and breadfruit are popular, as well as the starchy roots including yam, cassava, and sweet potatoes. Nut soups (with fruits or vegetables) and meat or fish stews are common and are usually thickened with vegetables such as spinach, kale, and pumpkin or nuts. Popular vegetables include okra, sweet peppers, and aubergines. Evaporated milk is taken in preference to cow's milk, and creamed coconut is often used for cooking. Most Afro-Caribbeans are Christians although those who are Rastafarian follow a largely vegetarian diet using no processed foods. The intake of sugar, salt, and fat tends to be high and sweet snacks are also very popular. However, the diet is generally sound because it is high in cereals, fruit, and vegetables and has modest amounts of protein and dairy products.

7. The Chinese diet

Most Chinese people in the United Kingdom originate from Hong Kong or South China. Northern Chinese peoples select wheat in the form of noodles, dumplings, and pancakes and some millet and sorghum as their staple foods. In southern China, rice is the main food although some wheat is also consumed. Cantonese foods are highly aromatic and contain delicate flavours and spices. Szechuan-style cooking is a feature of western China where dishes are hot and spicy, using chilli and black peppers. Many Chinese people will spend a lot of time selecting just the right ingredients often travelling great distances to get what they want. Fresh fruit, vegetables, and ingredients are bought and cooked in the same day. Traditionally, steamed noodles are served at breakfast. Soups, at lunch and dinner, are thin and clear and may be served with a garnish of raw vegetables (vegetables are rarely eaten raw except in this way). Fish, shellfish, and pork are commonly eaten. The desserts tend to be very rich, sticky, and oily.

The food is cooked quickly, in a stir-fry fashion, and with very little oil or fat. Eating customs include family meals where the family dig into large dishes of food with their fingers or chopsticks. The typical diet is quite sound nutritionally. It is low in fat and contains lots of fruit and vegetables. However, monosodium glutamate is consumed in large quantities and may lead to excessive intakes of sodium, raising a general health concern about the link between sodium intake and hypertension.

8. Summary

In this chapter we looked at the diets and the dietary customs of the Muslims, Hindus, Jews, Afro-Caribbeans and the Chinese. Their religion and culture strongly influence their diets, and there is a range of practical rules which must be observed when choosing or preparing food and when planning meals. There are also periods of fasting in some of these customs. A nurse's knowledge and understanding of the practices of these religious groups can encourage understanding and improve communication when interacting with these people.

Final Test for Module 4

Instructions

This section consists of 22 statements. Each one may be correct or incorrect. The answer required is either YES or NO. In your assessment of whether one of the 22 items is correct or not, you should base your answer only on the circumstances and facts given.

The questions are arranged in groups, in the order that the related topics occurred in the text. After ensuring that all the questions have been answered, check the results of the test yourself using the answers in the back of the book.

1. To maintain health, it is necessary to eat meat once a week.
2. Vegetarians do not eat meat or fish.
3. Vegans do not eat eggs, honey, milk or dairy products.
4. A lunch consisting of pea soup (without meat) and a jam-filled pancake is a well-balanced vegetarian meal.
5. A macrobiotic diet is part of a phi losophy in which the aim is to prolong life and improve the quality of life.
6. In a macrobiotic diet, meat, fish, milk and cheese are used sparingly.
7. According to anthroposophists, a meal that contains carrots, beetroot, celeriac, and swedes will have a positive influence on the nervous system and on the mental faculties.
8. In organic agriculture, no chemical weedkillers or artificial fertilisers are used.
9. Health foods often contain more saturated fat and less dietary fibre than ordinary food.
10. Muslims do not eat beef or veal.
11. Ramadan is the Islamic month of fasting when nothing should be eaten or drunk between sunrise and sunset.
12. Neither Jews nor Muslims will eat pork.
13. The cow is a sacred animal to Hindus.
14. Free range eggs have a higher nutritional value than battery eggs.
15. Jewish food laws allow pork to be served with a hot meal.
16. Jews do not use butter for frying meat, but they may use vegetable margarine instead.
17. Jews who live according to traditional customs normally use separate plates and cutlery for meat dishes from those used for dishes which contain dairy products.
18. Muslims do not drink alcohol.
19. Cereals in the Afro-Caribbean diet include corn, rice, oats, and wheat.
20. Afro-Caribbeans prefer cow's milk to evaporated milk.
21. Chinese people eat steamed noodles for breakfast.
22. Meat is the dominant feature of Chinese cooking.

References and further reading

British Nutrition Foundation, (1988) *Vegetarian Diets: Briefing Paper No 13.* British Nutrition Foundation, London.

California Dairy Council, (1981) *Asian Foods Guide for Teachers.* California Dairy Council, California.

Carlson E, Kipps M and Thomson J, (1983) Ethnic food habits. *Nutrition and Food Science,* No 6 (November/December), 21-22.

Currie C and Todd J, (1992) *Reports on the 1990 Scottish Health Behaviours in School Children Survey.* Research Unit in Health and Behavioural Change (RUHBC), Univeristy of Edinburgh, Edinburgh.

Deptartment of Health, (1993) *Ethnicity and Health: A Guide for the NHS.* HMSO, London.

Dobson S, (1991) *Transcultural Nursing.* Scutari Press, Harrow.

George M, (1994) *Accepting Differences.* Nursing Standard, 8, (18).

Henley A, (1982) *The Asian Patient in Hospital and at Home.* King Edward's Hospital Fund, London.

Henley A, (1982) *Asian Foods and Diets: A Training Pack.* National Extension College

Holt G, (1992) Investigating the diet of organic eaters. *Nutrition and Food Science,* No 6, (November/December), 13-16.

Karseras P and Hopkins E, (1987) *British Asians - Health in the Community.* John Wiley & Sons, Chichester.

Leininger M M, (1991) *Culture, Care Diversity and Universality: A Theory of Nursing.* National League for Nursing Press, New York.

Leininger M M, (1988) Leininger's theory of nursing: cultural care, diversity and universality. *Nursing Science Quarterly,* 1, (4), 152-160.

McNaught A, (1987) *Health Action and Ethnic Minorities.* National Community Health Resource/Bedford Square Press, London.

Mares P, Henley A and Baxter C (1985) *Health Care in Multiracial Britiain* Health Education Council/National Extension College.

Mikkelsen B, (1993) Organic foods in catering. *Nutrition and Food Science ,* No 3 ,(May/June), 24-26.

Sachs L, (1986) *Health Care Across Cultural Boundaries.* in *Migration and Health: Towards an Understanding of the Health Care Needs of Ethnic Minorities.* Colledge M et al (eds), WHO, Copenhagen.

Sanders T, (1979) *Vegan Nutrition.* The Vegan Society, Sussex.

Sussman V, (1978) *The Vegetarian Attitude: A Guide to a Healthful and Humane Diet.* Rodale Press, London.

Sutcliffe S, (1979) *Asian Families and Their Foods.* City of Bradford Metropolitan Council, Bradford.

Tan S, Wenlock R and Buss D, (1985) *Immigrant Foods: Second supplement to McCance and Widdowson's The Composition of Foods.* HMSO, London.

Weller B, (1991) Nursing in a multicultural world. *Nursing Standard,* 5, 31-32.

Module 5

DIET AND THE TREATMENT OF DISEASE

Introduction to Module 5

In the treatment and management of disease, maintaining the correct diet may be an essential requirement. A diet prescribed for medical reasons may differ from our average eating habits in quantity, consistency and content, and adhering to it may mean a drastic change in the patient's lifestyle, with an alteration of the regular dietary pattern. In addition, the patient's circumstances may not always be conducive to maintaining such a diet.

When a patient is following a diet, nursing staff can play an important role in monitoring the intake of food and drink and providing guidance. Patients should be helped to accept and understand the importance of maintaining the regime, since failure to adhere to a diet (or too strict an interpretation of its requirements) may simply be the result of a lack of information about why it is needed, or inadequate knowledge about the options and variations which may exist within it.

The nursing staff, in conjunction with the dietitian, should also be able to answer any questions that arise from the patient when a diet has been prescribed. If they see problems arising, they should alert the relevant staff and liaise with the patient to find a solution. Nearly all diets form part of a therapy, though some may be used to aid diagnosis.

The therapeutic diet

1. Introduction

This chapter explains the processes involved in giving dietary advice to an individual. It also explains the meanings of some of the terms and expressions commonly used in dietetics.

Diet can be an important element in the treatment of disease. A diet high in dietary fibre, for example, can correct certain bowel conditions, and a diet rich in protein can improve the physical condition of a seriously ill patient and thus speed recovery. A high proportion of the meals prepared in hospital kitchens may be for specialised, therapeutic diets.

Learning outcomes

After studying this chapter the student should be able to:
- explain in her own words the meanings of the terms *therapeutic diet, dietary prescription* and *dietary advice;*
- describe how a patient can obtain dietary advice;
- name the three different classifications of diet, giving an example of each;
- understand and use the generally accepted abbreviations for common diets;
- explain why following a diet may have an impact on many people's lives;
- describe the role of the nursing staff in counselling a patient on a diet.

2. What is a diet?

The word *diet* can be defined as a pattern of nutrition which has, for medical reasons, to meet certain specifications for the benefit of a particular person. This means that a diet must be of an individual nature, precisely matched to meet the requirements and preferences of the patient. A diet is also prescribed for medical reasons, so adherence to kosher or vegetarian food, for example, cannot be classified as a diet in the proper sense of the word.

A diet is compiled by a dietitian, to whom the patient has been referred by a doctor. This usually involves a standard set of procedures:
- the doctor sends written instruction to the dietitian containing medical information about the patient (including the diagnosis);

- the dietitian then compiles a diet based on the *dietary prescription* (the specific requirements which the diet should meet);
- The dietary prescription is then translated into *dietary advice* by dietitian and patient together. This dietary advice will comprise a number of practical guidelines including *nutrients* and actual *foodstuffs* for a diet which, as far as possible, take the circumstances and eating habits of the patient into account;
- The patient's dietary history compiled by the dietitian, is one of the important starting points. Figure 5.1.1 shows the stages involved.

3. Classification of diets

In the past, diets were often named after the disease or the diseased organ which they were intended to cure (such as the *gastric diet*), or after the person who developed them (such as the *Sippy cure*). Medically speaking, names like these do not sufficiently reflect the essence of the diet. Furthermore, it is considered unwise to emphasise the disease or the affected organ in diet nomenclature. Currently, the names of diets reflect the way in which they differ from everyday dietary patterns, though these characteristics are, of course, related to the group of symptoms in question.

The therapeutic diets can be classified into three groups:
- *Nutrient-rich or nutrient-restricted diets*
  These are diets in which one or more nutrients have to be included in set amounts. Examples include a diet rich in dietary fibre or a sodium-restricted diet.
- *Nutrient-free diets*
  These are exclusion diets in which a specific nutrient is excluded completely. Examples include the gluten-free diet or a diet which excludes benzoic acid (a preservative).
- *Altered consistency diets*
  In these diets, the consistency of the food has been altered, and examples include a liquidised or a minced diet.

There are a number of standard abbreviations used in notations for diets, and some of the most common are listed in Figure 5.1.2.

Figure 5.1.1
The process involved in arriving at dietary advice

Doctor	Doctor and/or dietitian	Dietitian
diagnosis	dietary prescription (in nutrients)	dietary advice (in foodstuffs)
example: obesity	restricted energy diet	practical information about diet, precisely matched to the requirements and preferences of individual patients

Figure 5.1.2
Abbreviations of dietetic terminology

Abbreviation   *Term*

ENE	energy
PRO	protein
glut	gluten
CHO	carbohydrates
lac	lactose
sac	saccharin
DF	dietary fibre
pufa	polyunsaturated fatty acids
chol	cholesterol
Na	sodium
K	potassium
DM	diabetes mellitus
light	semi-fluid diet

Study activity 1

a. Do vegetarian diets constitute a therapeutic diet? Explain your answer.
b. Have you ever been on a diet yourself? If so, what did you think of the experience?

4. Dietary counselling

Adhering to a diet may involve a significant change in everyday life. Habits which have been established over a long period and which have become an integral part of a person's life may have to be changed. Even when the diet is carefully adapted to the patient's preferences and is varied and well prepared, it may still represent a long-term limitation on the patient's freedom. In addition, the benefits of the diet may not always immediately be noticeable.

It is fairly common, therefore, for diets not to be strictly adhered to. There may be a number of reasons for this, such as failure to understand or to remember advice or instructions about the diet, lack of support from family and friends, politeness when dining with others or the temptations encountered in shop windows, in restaurants and through advertising. Diets may also be ignored during special occasions like parties and other social functions, and at certain periods like holidays. The difficulties or inconvenience of always preparing food that complies with the diet may also be a factor.

In institutional health care the nursing staff can play an important role in dietary counselling, and any signs suggesting that a patient is having problems keeping to a diet can be acted upon quickly.

Patients may need advice and information about their diets and, wherever possible, the nurse and patient should work together to solve problems, keeping the ward sister or dietitian informed as necessary. Other patients or support groups may also lend encouragement, particularly where the diet has to be maintained for a long time.

Study activity 2

Following a major heart attack, Mr Edwards, who is 40 years old and married, has been convalescing for a week in the cardiology ward of a hospital. He is a bakery manager and had been feeling tired and short of breath before the heart attack, which was probably caused by his weight (he is 178 cm tall (5 ft 10 in) and weighs 100 kg (15 st 10 lb)). He is very worried about having another attack and will do all he can to prevent one. The cardiologist thinks he should lose some weight and prescribes a low energy diet. He also advised Mr Edwards to stop smoking, and this advice was acted on immediately.

Ideally, Mr Edwards wants to lose 20 kg (3 st). However, he has pointed out that, while he has no problem adhering to the diet when he is in the hospital, where the food is specially prepared for him and the staff are all very supportive, the difficulties will start on his return home and if and when he returns to work.

a. Why will it be so difficult for Mr Edwards to maintain his diet at home?
b. How can consultation with a dietitian help him before he leaves the hospital?

Study activity 3

    a. Nursing staff are expected to provide dietary advice regularly. What kind of advice do patients require most?

    b. Nursing staff can greatly support the work of the dietitian. In which phase of the problem-solving process will their support be particularly useful? Explain using an example (refer to Module 1, Chapter 2).

5. Summary

Many of the meals provided within the Health Service are specially prepared for patients following a therapeutic diet. This chapter has explained the meanings of the most common terms in dietetics, and described how dietary advice is formulated. Maintaining a diet may involve radical changes for patients, and for their families, so guidance by the nursing staff can be very important both for informing and motivating patients.

The staff can also help to teach patients about handling specially prepared food. Support can be given by informing patients clearly about the diet, being alert to problems and trying to solve them in consultation with a doctor and dietitian wherever necessary.

Diet and illness

1. Introduction

Illness can be accompanied by a number of problems such as pain, stress, and fatigue which may cause loss of appetite. When the illness is acute and of short duration (such as influenza) loss of appetite is not a major problem. With febrile illnesses it is more important to drink adequately than to eat.

During a long-term illness, however, maintaining a nutritional and well-balanced diet becomes extremely important. This is because, despite any lack of appetite, a patient maintaining a healthy diet will usually feel better and recover more easily and quickly, and an appropriate diet will also aid absorption of medicines.

This chapter examines dietary management during the more serious long-term illnesses.

Learning outcomes

After studying this chapter the student should be able to:
- name ten different factors that can cause loss of appetite;
- describe the consequences of minimal food intake over a long period of time;
- explain the sort of care which is important for patients who have lost their appetite, and illustrate this with an example;
- list six recommendations for patients who have lost their appetites;
- explain why a meal for someone with a depressed appetite should not contain much fat, especially non-emulsified fat;
- plan a lunch and a dinner suitable for someone with little appetite;
- list five situations which can lead to undernourishment;
- give two characteristics of a diet suitable for an undernourished patient;
- understand the ways in which an undernourished patient's daily menu can be improved;
- explain the interaction between food and medication;
- explain the implications of an impending medical examination or operation with regard to food intake;

– explain how patients are reintroduced to food after surgery involving a general anaesthetic;

– explain why a fluid balance chart has to be maintained after surgery involving a general anaesthetic.

2. Loss of appetite

a. Causes of loss of appetite

When someone is ill, several physical and mental factors can lead to loss of appetite. These include pain, stress, fever, fear, fatigue, infections and the need to remain in bed. Some medications and treatments, such as the chemotherapy and radio-therapy given to cancer patients, can also suppress the appetite or cause nausea. Surroundings can also play an important role. A hospital or nursing home may not be the most pleasant place to eat, and a fellow patient or resident who eats noisily or retches during meals may severely depress the appetite of other patients.

Case study

Mrs Campbell is 78 years old and has recently been admitted to the obser-vation ward of a nursing home where, at five o'clock every afternoon, the dining-room table is laid for tea. All the resi-dents have allocated seats at the table, where they sit every day.

Mrs Campbell is kind and helpful, and usually chats amicably with the other residents, but during meals she remains silent, trying not to glance up at the other residents. This is because she can see her neighbour dribbling saliva from the side of his mouth; furthermore, the man sitting opposite her constantly licks his spoon noisily. Mrs Campbell finds all this has a negative effect on her appetite.

Mrs Campbell is fortunate in that she is still able to maintain a neat appear-ance, and she eats in a well-mannered and socially acceptable fashion. Never-

theless, the staff will not allow her to eat alone: 'It's much nicer to eat together in the dining-room', they tell her.

Study activity 1

Can you list a number of factors that you have encountered on a ward or in an institution which might spoil someone's appetite? Suggest some ways in which these factors could be prevented or elimi-nated.

b. Consequences of a reduced appetite

It is not a major problem if a patient eats little or nothing for a short period of time, especially if his or her dietary status was good before the onset of the illness. It is very important, however, that a patient drinks sufficient to prevent dehydration. This is particularly important when fever, vomiting, diarrhoea or perspiration oc-curs.

The consequences can be serious, how-ever, if the appetite remains poor for an extended period. This can often be ob-served in patients with cancer, depression, or kidney disease, in alcoholics, and the mentally handicapped (particularly those who also have impaired muscular control).

Figure 5.2.1

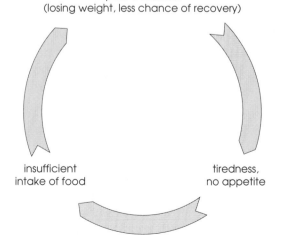

poor condition
(losing weight, less chance of recovery)

insufficient
intake of food

tiredness,
no appetite

A patient's nutritional status can seriously deteriorate if insufficient food is eaten over a long period. The chance of a full recovery declines, wounds take longer to heal, and the risk of infection increases. There is also a greater risk of bedsores in bedridden patients. The patient may become tired and listless, leading to further loss of appetite, thus creating a vicious circle (Figure 5.2.1).

The introduction of a specially formulated diet may improve the patient's condition and break this vicious circle, though there are concerns that the changes taking place in the NHS may compromise the provision of nutritious meals (Figure 5.2.2).

Figure 5.2.2
The Herald 8/4/94

Starvation in our hospitals

Alan MacDermid

...A recent study, by dietician Janet McWhirter and consultant physician Chris Pennington, looked at the nutritional status of 500 patients, evenly divided among general surgery, general medicine, respiratory, orthopaedic and elderly care. The tale they tell is one that could well be found in many big hospitals, and is less a reflection on the standard of cuisine at Ninewells than a failure by clinical staff to recognise or look for the signs of malnutrition.

It must say something about the state of the country that 200 out of the 500 were undernourished when they came in the first place, even allowing that undernourished people are more likely to end up in hospital.

...The mean weight loss amounted to some 5.4%, but it was those who came in thinnest who lost more weight; a quarter who had been mildly undernourished became moderately undernourished, and 37% who had been moderately undernourished were severely undernourished when they left.

Clearly this needn't have happened – those who had been specifically sent to the hospital for nutritional support fared better, and showed a gain in weight. But fewer than half of the 200 patients who came in malnourished had any information on their case notes about their nutritional state.

The gap McWhirter and Pennington have spotted is one of awareness on the part of those assessing patients for referral.

...No patient need starve in hospital. So how does it happen? Perhaps they are victims of the streamlined efficiency of the modern hospital.

John Garrow, Rank Professor of Human Nutrition at Bart's London, comments on the Ninewells findings: "It is administrative changes that have made it more difficult to ensure that ordinary patients get proper meals. Before the recent reforms, if a patient who had been fasted for blood tests in the morning and returned from radiology at 2.30pm, having missed lunch, the ward sister could provide him with scrambled egg on toast prepared in the ward kitchen.

"In most hospitals this is no longer possible; catering services are supplied on a tightly budgeted contract, and extra, informal meals require a referral to the dietician. "High hygiene standards have the result that nurses are not allowed to prepare any cooked food in most ward kitchens.

"So, instead of getting scrambled eggs, the patient will probably have to wait until his next evening meal, having fasted for 24 hours. The same events may occur the next day. No wonder malnourished patients often lose weight in hospital."

c. Caring for patients with a depressed appetite

It is important that the staff responsible for a patient's daily care are alert to notice any loss of appetite, since they are the people in the best position to observe which problems influence eating and drinking behaviour. When a patient suffers from stress, fear or fatigue, it is advisable to talk it over with him. The patient must be given the opportunity to rest before meals, and ample time to eat the meals.

A quiet atmosphere during meal times may help, and it is always advisable to consider the patient's wishes about where, what, and how he wants to eat. The nursing staff may encourage a patient to eat and drink by talking about the importance of a nutritional and well-balanced diet and, where necessary, they can assist the patient with eating and drinking. A dietitian can be called in to formulate the correct diet.

d. General advice for treating patients with a depressed appetite

- The appetite can be stimulated by serving half a cup of broth or a small glass of fruit juice half an hour before the meal;
- Large servings can lead to a depressed appetite being lost completely. Serve smaller meals more often (five or six small meals a day rather than three large ones). If the patient tends to feel hungry during the night, this opportunity should be used and food can be left on the bedside table or locker if necessary;
- Food that looks appetising and smells and tastes good will stimulate the appetite. In a hospital or nursing home, this is the catering department's task, but the nursing staff can help by ensuring that meals are served on clean plates and that tables or trays are laid out neatly and attractively. They should also try to take the patient's likes and dislikes into consideration, serving an alternative when a dish the patient dislikes is on the menu;
- The food should not be too greasy, as rich food stays in the stomach for a long time and therefore suppresses hunger. It is recommended that the food contains emulsified fat, which is distributed throughout the food in small particles, since fats in this form are more easily digestible. Emulsified fats can be found in foods such as butter, margarine, cream, full cream milk, egg yolk, and mayonnaise. Fatty meats and fried dishes contain non-emulsified fats, and so are more difficult to digest. The fat in gravy is also non-emulsified, because butter and margarine lose their emulsified form when they are heated.

Example

- A meal consisting of fatty meat, potatoes, rich gravy and cauliflower and cheese sauce contains a lot of fat, most of which is non-emulsified and may be rather heavy on the stomach;
- Finely chopped food, stew, mashed potatoes, and porridge are easier to digest. Dishes like these are also easier to eat because they do not require much chewing. For similar reasons, fruit juice and stewed fruit are often preferred to ordinary fruit;
- Drinking enough fluid (at least 1.5 litres per day) can improve a patient's appetite by allowing waste products to be eliminated more easily. If these products build up in the bloodstream they can induce feelings of nausea;
- Fizzy drinks and whipped cream are very filling. It is better to use unwhipped cream in desserts, soups, sauces, coffee and other drinks;
- For slow eaters, the meal might become cold and unappetising before it is finished and some means of keeping the food warm may be a solution;
- Physical activity, when appropriate, can improve a patient's appetite.

Study activity 2

A 62-year-old lady has been a patient in a psychiatric hospital for a few weeks. She is a small, slight woman and normally good-natured. She feels fine physically, but her appetite has recently declined. Breakfast is the only meal she can manage. She often eats only half her lunch, and has just a slice of bread in the evening. At around noon today she had the following:
- a small bowl of soup
- a helping of shepherd's pie
- 2 spoonfuls of gravy
- 1 helping of chocolate dessert with whipped cream.

She does not want any supper at all in the evening.

Try to explain why she refused to eat at all in the evening.

How could this problem be solved?

Study activity 3

a. Comment on the following statements:
- A malnourished person should take increased amounts of protein, such as large servings of meat;
- Broth strengthens malnourished patients;
- Variety is the spice of a diet.
b. In Module 2, Chapter 1, the visible characteristics of malnourishment were described. List at least five of these characteristics.

3. Malnourishment

Malnourishment, or the threat of malnourishment, is particularly prevalent in the chronically ill, but it can also occur after major surgery or in patients suffering from serious burns. When major surgery is impending, extra nutrients are usually given beforehand to promote rapid recovery after the operation. It is important to start feeding the patient as soon as possible after the operation, by mouth if possible, but by parenteral feeding (tube-feeding) if necessary.

A high energy and high protein diet can help to improve a patient's condition and alleviate any symptoms of under-nutrition. The patient will then feel better, recovery will be accelerated, and the vicious circle illustrated in Figure 5.2.1 can be broken.

a. Energy and protein
To improve a patient's nutritional status, meals have to satisfy the following conditions:
- They must be high in energy. The basis of the diet should be wholesome food, supplemented with additional carbohydrates (sugar and starch) and emulsified fats. Too much fat should be avoided as it reduces the appetite;
- They must be rich in protein. Adding extra protein to a diet is only useful, however, if there is enough energy already present in the form of carbohydrates and fat. If there is insufficient energy, the protein in the food will be used as fuel instead of a building material;
- They must contain vitamins and minerals in the quantities appropriate to the patient's requirements. For example, extra vitamin C, vitamin A and zinc promote the healing of wounds, and additional calcium and vitamin D will assist in the repair of fractured bones.

Undernourished patients often suffer from loss of appetite, and all the suggestions mentioned previously on encouraging the patient to eat will be instrumental in alleviating the problem.

A diet can be made richer in energy in the following ways:
- By using full fat dairy products such as full cream milk, full fat yoghurt and cream cheese;
- By giving extra snacks and drinks such as milk shakes, custard, cottage cheese with fruit, cocoa, fruit juice or ready-prepared energy drinks (which are also

rich in protein, vitamins and minerals);

– By adding butter or margarine to mashed potatoes, vegetables or porridge, or by spreading them generously on bread;

– By using glucose polymers instead of normal sugar. These are not as sweet as ordinary sugars but contain an equivalent amount of energy, so they can be used in greater quantities to obtain the same level of sweetness (see also Figure 5.6.2, in Chapter 6 of this module);

– By adding unwhipped cream to drinks such as coffee, and to liquid dishes such as desserts, custard, porridge, yoghurt, soups, sauces, and mashed potatoes.

A diet can be made richer in protein by:
– using generous quantities of cheese or meat in sandwiches;
– serving cheese snacks between meals;
– using meat in stews and salads;
– serving custard or porridge instead of sandwiches or toast;
– serving cottage cheese, which has a high protein content (a generous spoonful of cottage cheese contains as much protein as a glass of milk);
– making coffee with hot milk instead of water;
– adding a powdered protein preparation to liquid or semi-solid foods such as milk, yoghurt, custard, porridge, white coffee, and milk shakes (see also Figure 5.6.2, in Chapter 6 of this module).

If extra protein is required the following can be served each day:
– 1 or 2 pints of milk, yoghurt, or custard dessert;
– 2 pieces of cheese or 1 egg;
– 150 g of lean meat, fish, or chicken (used as fillings in sandwiches, for example).

Study activity 4

An 81-year-old man has recently been admitted to hospital with symptoms of Parkinson's disease. He cannot walk very well, and he finds it very difficult to talk. In recent months, the tremor in his arms has become more marked and his appetite has deteriorated. He has lost a lot of weight over a short period of time, and now weighs 64 kg (10 st 3 lb) and he is 181 cm (6 ft) tall.

a. What general advice should be given about this patient's diet?

b. Yesterday his menu was as follows:
   Breakfast
   1 slice of white bread with margarine
   1 rasher of bacon
   tea
   Elevenses
   white coffee with sugar
   Lunch
   1 small bowl of soup
   1 very small serving of meat with a potato and sliced carrot
   1 small bowl of rice pudding
   Tea
   1 cup of tea
   Dinner
   1 slice of white bread with margarine and jam
   1 slice of Madeira cake spread with margarine
   1 cup of tea
   Supper
   white coffee with sugar
   1 glass of fruit juice
   What would you change in this menu? Try to plan a more appropriate daily menu using ordinary food.

c. The patient's menu was changed using ordinary food, but his condition does not appear to have improved significantly. What kinds of special dietary products could be used, either for his main meals or as snacks between meals?

Figure 5.2.3
Recipe for milk shake

Ingredients
1 glass of milk
2 tablespoons of ice-cream
4 tablespoons of fruit purée (such as banana, strawberry, or peach purée) or fruit juice
a dash of cream

Method
Place all the ingredients in a bowl and whisk together.
Pour the drink into a tall glass.

b. Diet, medical examinations and surgery
For a short period before undergoing a medical examination or surgery, a patient is often served food that differs from the food he or she normally eats, or else no food at all. As the dietary preparations (or 'preps') preceding medical examinations and operations differ according to the hospital concerned, and are changed frequently, there is little point in listing them in this publication. However, the duration of the diet must always be adjusted according to the patient's condition, and should take account of factors such as nausea and vomiting.

Briefly, the diet prescribed before a medical examination or operation usually consists of food which can be easily digested. Consequently, it is often low in fat and it may be of a specified consistency (usually liquid).

On the day of the examination or operation, the patient will be served either a light breakfast or nothing at all. If a general anaesthetic is to be used, the stomach must be empty. On the other hand, the prerequisite for some medical examinations is additional fluid intake.

Following an examination or surgery using local anaesthetic, a normal diet can be resumed immediately. Following a general anaesthetic, however, return to solid foods must be gradual, beginning

with a given quantity of water every hour and the progressing to a diet of liquid and finely minced food and then to light meals before eventually returning to a normal diet. The reintroduction of solid food, however, depends on gastrointestinal activity, and flatulence and defecation are indications of this.

It is very important to keep track of a patient's fluid balance after surgery, since the fluid intake must reach levels sufficient to flush out the waste products from the body which build up as a result of the operation.

c. Diet and medicine
Since most patients are taking at least one form of medication, the interaction between food and medication is always an important consideration. Research has shown that there is a two-way influence between the interaction of food and drugs in the body.

The following examples illustrate the types of interactions which may take place:
–   Iron preparations (used in the treatment of anaemia) should not be taken in combination with dairy products or other products high in protein, because protein hinders the resorption of iron in the body. The iron will be more easily resorbed in combination with fruit juice;
–   Even small amounts of alcohol will affect the efficacy of many medicines, such as antidepressants. The interaction can seriously impair the patient's response to the drug;
–   Some diuretics cause excess minerals to be excreted in the urine and this can result in loss of calcium. Increasing fruit consumption (or drinking fruit juice) helps to remedy this;
–   A number of medicines tend to dull the sense of taste. Examples include drugs for patients with Parkinson's disease (such as levodopa), some antihypertensives (such as captopril), some medicines for severe rheumatoid arthritis (such as penicillamine) and some

of the chemotherapeutics used in the treatment of cancer. If a patient's appetite deteriorates as a result of using these medicines, one possible solution may be the serving of smaller meals more frequently;

– Some medicines can cause constipation. Examples of these include iron preparations, antihypertensives, cough lozenges containing codeine and painkillers such as morphine;

– Sometimes specific medicines require that a particular diet be followed. For instance, when MAOI (monoamine oxidase inhibitors) are administered to treat depression, the amino acid tyramine will not be broken down sufficiently and will accumulate. This is potentially lethal if there is a rise in blood pressure. Patients taking these medicines will, therefore, be put on a tyramine-restricted diet which means reducing the intake of coffee, chocolate, cola, beer, wine, herring, broad beans, cold meat and ripe cheeses such as Camembert, Brie, and Gruyère;

– A number of medicines can cause thirst. One example is lithium, which is used in the treatment of manic-depressive psychoses;

– Long-term use of anticonvulsants can cause a lack of vitamin D;

– Long-term use of antibiotics can restrict the body's supply of vitamin K. This is because vitamin K is produced by bacteria that are present naturally in our intestines. Since antibiotics are likely to inhibit growth of some of the intestinal flora, production of vitamin K consequently becomes restricted.

These examples show that not only does diet influence the efficacy of medicines but medicines influence the nutritional status of the patient by suppressing the appetite or the resorption of nutrients in the body. Unfortunately, in practice, insufficient attention is paid to food–drug interaction.

4. Summary

Loss of appetite can be caused by a number of physical and psychological factors. If the appetite remains suppressed for a long period of time, the patient's nutritional status will deteriorate and this can have serious consequences. It may reduce the capacity for recovery and increase the risk of complications.

The care of patients suffering from loss of appetite has been discussed in this chapter and some recommendations for improving the appetite have been given.

In a patient who is not receiving adequate nutrition or who is likely to become undernourished, nutritional status can be improved by following a high energy, high protein diet. A number of methods of increasing the energy and protein content of a diet were examined, using both ordinary food and special dietary products. Dietary preparation for medical examinations and surgery have been covered briefly, and the chapter ended by introducing food–drug interactions which must be taken into account when planning a diet.

Diet and diabetes mellitus

1. Introduction

In Britain, diabetes is known to affect approximately 1 to 1.5% of the population. However, there are probably a great many sufferers who have not yet been diagnosed as suffering from the condition. Diabetes is prevalent in people over 65, amongst whom the incidence rises to around 10%.

Obviously, it is quite a shock to learn from your GP that you have diabetes mellitus because it will have a major impact on the rest of your life. It is, therefore, essential that the health care workers you come into contact with can offer understanding and appropriate counselling as well as adequate information.

Learning outcomes

After studying this chapter, the student should be able to:
- list two short-term and two long-term aims of the treatment of diabetes mellitus;
- explain the difference between the two forms of diabetes mellitus (type I and type II);
- outline how the type of therapy affects the diet;
- explain why it is so important for a diabetic patient to eat regularly;
- explain why patients suffering from diabetes mellitus should restrict their intake of saturated fats and choose unsaturated fats instead;
- describe how a normal level of glucose in the blood can be maintained;
- describe the correct dietary action and dietary care to take when hypoglycaemia develops;
- name two kinds of sweetener suitable for the diabetic patient;
- give one benefit and one disadvantage of energy-free or intense sweeteners;
- demonstrate the variety of food which is possible within the constraints of a diabetic diet;
- use the carbohydrate exchange list to substitute one meal with another which contains the same amount of carbohydrates;

- list the factors which a diabetic should take into consideration when selecting a diet to have a positive influence on the blood glucose level;
- explain how the insulin pump and the insulin injection pen have different advantages with respect to the diet of diabetic patients.

Case study

Mrs Richardson is a 75-year-old woman who was admitted to the surgical ward of a hospital a week ago. She is small, 158 cm (5 ft 2 in) tall, and weighs 70.2 kg (11 st 2 lb). Five years ago, when she had been suffering from intense thirst, itchiness, tiredness, and polyuria (excessive excretion of urine), she was diagnosed by her GP as having diabetes mellitus. The GP prescribed a diet in conjunction with pills.

However, as a result of her condition, one of Mrs Richardson's toes has become necrotic and requires amputation. She is in severe pain and cries from time to time. Since diagnosis of her condition, she has found her diet difficult to maintain. Her husband and children visit regularly, always bringing something for her to eat.

Study activity 1

a. Why does Mrs Richardson have problems maintaining her diet?

b. If she continually fails to maintain her diet, what are the possible consequences?

c. What do you think about family members bringing food for her during visiting hours?

d. What is your opinion of Mrs Richardson's weight?

2. Diabetes mellitus

Diabetes mellitus can be defined as a chronic disease characterised by the body's insufficient production of insulin or insufficient functioning of insulin. This causes metabolic disturbance. Symptoms include a high level of glucose concentration in the blood and excretion of glucose in the urine.

a. The two forms of diabetes mellitus

Two forms of diabetes mellitus can be distinguished:

Type I (or *insulin-dependent diabetes mellitus*) is a form in which no insulin, or very little, is produced. This form often appears at an early age, though it can also occur later in life.

Case study

Jean Williams, who works in a small grocery store, is 18 years old, 167 cm (5 ft 6 in) tall and weighs 54 kg (8 st 10 lb). Recently, she has begun to feel thirsty all the time, having a drink at least every hour whilst at work, and she seemed to be going to the toilet frequently. She began to eat increasing amounts, and her mother became especially worried by the way she was losing weight in spite of her increasing appetite, and also because she was constantly tired.

Her doctor diagnosed diabetes and referred her to a hospital specialist, who saw her as an outpatient. He prescribed insulin and she was referred to a dietitian who advised her on a suitable diet. At first, Jean was very confused and found it difficult to come to terms with the fact that she was diabetic, but one of the nurses who specialised in diabetes recommended that she contact an ex-patient she knew who was about the same age, and had had diabetes since she was 13. Jean found a lot of help and support from her contact with this girl and she gradually accepted her condition, learning how to handle her diet and how to inject insulin.

Type II (non-insulin-dependent diabetes mellitus, or maturity-onset diabetes) is the form which affects 85-90% of diabetics. People with this form do produce some insulin, but not enough. Treatment includes a diet, which may be supported by oral hypoglycaemic agents (which lower the level of glucose in the blood by activating the patient's own production of insulin) or by insulin injections. This form is seen mostly in people over 40, and many of the patients are overweight (as in the example in section 2).

Diabetes Type II is often diagnosed only after complications have occurred and is usually detected accidentally during routine tests or investigations.

b. The treatment of diabetes mellitus

The treatment of diabetes mellitus is aimed at maintaining normal blood glucose concentration (between 6 and 9 mmol/litre). Thus, it attempts to prevent hypoglycaemia (where the blood glucose concentration is too low, under 3 mmol/litre) and hyperglycaemia (where the blood glucose concentration is too high, over 10 mmol/litre).

A second and equally important aim is the prevention or postponement of long-term symptoms. A high proportion of diabetics suffer from degeneration of the blood vessels, nerves, kidneys and eyes, caused partly by high levels of glucose in the blood. The risk of such complications increases when a person has been a diabetic for a long time, but it has been established that patients who have administered correct amounts of insulin are less at risk. Complications may still arise with such patients, however, and it is likely that factors other than glucose level are also implicated, such as elevations in serum cholesterol levels.

A central part of the therapy used to achieve these aims is the implementation of a diet adapted to the individual patient. The diet and insulin injections will be adjusted as far as possible to ensure optimal compatibility with the patient's lifestyle.

The therapies available for the two types of diabetes can be summarised as follows:

In type I diabetes, the level of glucose in the blood is usually controlled by diet in combination with insulin injections.

In type II diabetes, the level of glucose in the blood is usually controlled in one of two ways: by diet only or by diet in combination with oral medication.

Diabetics of both types are treated as outpatients, wherever possible, when determining the amount of insulin needed, so that the disruption to their daily routine is minimal.

3. Diet for diabetics

The diet is the cornerstone in the treatment of diabetes mellitus.

The diabetic diet is essentially the kind of healthy diet which everybody should aim for, but it has additional criteria which have to be met: it should prevent too much fluctuation in the level of glucose in the blood, and it should attain, or maintain, a body weight appropriate to the individual. Too much body fat reduces the effectiveness of the insulin. Consequently, weight loss is often the fundamental aim when planning the diet for a type II patient since these patients are usually overweight. When such a patient attains an appropriate body weight, the body needs far less insulin, with the result that medication can be reduced or even stopped.

a. Characteristics of a diabetic diet

A diabetic diet has the following characteristics:
- The meals must be regular. As well as three main meals per day, three or four snacks must be eaten between meals so that glucose from the food reaches the blood steadily and there is less risk of sudden peaks in the glucose level (Figures 5.3.1a and b). Eating regular meals also allows the insulin (whether

it is naturally present, injected, or taken as oral hypoglycaemic agents) to metabolise the glucose more efficiently.

– There should be a balanced distribution of carbohydrates. Carbohydrates should be taken in small and regular amounts over six or seven meals throughout the day to avoid fluctuations in blood glucose levels which would otherwise arise.

Carbohydrates are preferably given in the form of starch and dietary fibre, in foods such as bread, potatoes, pulses and fresh fruit. Foods rich in dietary fibre are particularly recommended because carbohydrates from such foods are absorbed into the blood more slowly. The dietary fibre slows down glucose absorption and, as a result, slows down the increase in the blood glucose level. Therefore, it is better to recommend wholemeal bread rather than white bread, and fruit instead of fruit juice.

– The daily energy intake from the diet is suited to the patient's needs. The starting points for determining the amount of energy needed are the patient's dietary history, body weight, and pattern of activity. Someone who exercises, participates in regular sports activities or whose job entails heavy lifting will need more energy than someone who leads a sedentary life. On the other hand, an overweight person will often be prescribed an energy-restricted diabetic diet.

– The amount of saturated fat is restricted and is partly substituted by unsaturated fat. This is because diabetics are at greater risk of developing cardiovascular disease, and too much fatty food may also hinder the activity of insulin. Dairy products and fatty meats should preferably be replaced by low fat alternatives such as oils, vegetable margarine and diet margarine, which have a beneficial effect on the cardiovascular system.

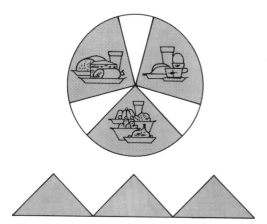

Figure 5.3.1a
Level of glucose in the blood when eating three large main meals a day

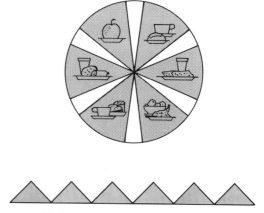

Figure 5.3.1b
Level of glucose in the blood when eating three small main meals a day with three snacks in between

Figure 5.3.2
Diabetic foods

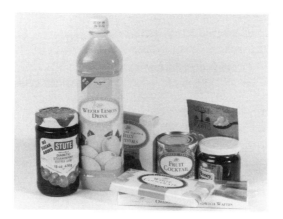

Study activity 2

How can a diabetic attain normoglycaemia (a constant normal blood glucose level)?

When compiling a diet, the dietitian will consider the habits, preferences and capabilities of the patient whenever possible. The less the diet diverges from the person's former eating habits, the more acceptable it will be and the easier it will be to follow.

The four characteristics of a diabetic diet listed above can be seen in the example shown in Figure 5.3.3.

b. Differences between type I and type II diets

The characteristics of the diabetic diet listed above apply to both types of diabetes mellitus, but the individual dietary considerations may differ depending on the type of medication prescribed (see Figure 5.3.5).

4. The diabetic diet past and present

The diabetic diet used to be much stricter than it is now, and it was thought that precise timing of the meals was of crucial importance. However, no one has the same routine from day to day, and minor changes in eating schedules are consequently now regarded as acceptable. The diabetic no longer needs to weigh each item of food, although the size of the portions should still be carefully regulated. Approximate measures such as a third of a plate of vegetables, for example, or a medium-

sized apple, will normally be adequate. Sometimes, however, with foodstuffs rich in carbohydrates which can be difficult to estimate, such as rice, pasta, or pulses, it may still be prudent to weigh the portions initially, until the patient becomes familiar with portion sizes.

Ideas about the use of sugar have also changed over the past few years, and this is covered more fully in Section 6.

5. Varying the diet

Apart from basic dietary advice, a diabetic will require information on how daily meals can be varied. Understanding how this can be done will help diabetics to feel more comfortable in various social situations, as they will then be able to make appropriate food choices from buffets and set menus at parties and other social functions. There are several exchange lists that can be used for the purpose, and an example is given in Appendix 2. A list of this kind makes it possible to substitute parts of meals while keeping the amount of carbohydrate the same. Extensive lists are published by the British Diabetic Association.

An example of the use of an exchange list is given below:

One small slice of bread (10 grams of carbohydrates) with cheese or ham can be replaced by:

two crackers with cheese or ham

or a 150 ml bowl of porridge without sugar

or two small digestive biscuits.

Figure 5.3.3
Diabetic diet

Example of a diabetic diet (Type I, normal body weight)	Carbohydrate content (grams)	Possible alternative meals
Breakfast 1 slice of wholemeal bread with low fat diet margarine low fat cheese or lean meat 1 glass of low fat milk tea without sugar	30	*Breakfast* 1 slice of fruit loaf with low-fat diet margarine 2 crackers with peanut butter 1 glass of buttermilk tea without sugar
Morning Snack coffee with milk 1 slice of wholemeal bread with low fat diet margarine low fat cheese or lean meat 1 glass of low fat milk	20	*Morning Snack* 1 small slice of cake 1 cup of cocoa made with semi-skimmed milk (add sweetener if desired)
Lunch clear soup 1 portion of lean meat 3 potatoes chicken gravy generous helping of vegetables vegetable salad (optional)	50	*Lunch* tomato soup chicken biryani (two serving spoons of cooked rice, breast and mixed vegetables) cucumber 1 helping dessert (with sugar)
Tea tea without sugar 1 cracker with low fat diet margarine low fat meat 1 piece of fruit (e.g. 1 apple)	20	*Tea* tea without sugar 1 digestive biscuit 1 plate of cherries
Dinner 3 slices of wholemeal bread with low fat diet margarine 2 portions of a cheese or meat product 1 portion of jam or marmalade (with sugar) vegetable salad tea without sugar	60	*Dinner* 1 wholemeal roll 2 crackers with low fat diet margarine cheese and cucumber ham and tomato lemon curd (with sugar) tea without sugar
Supper coffee or tea with milk 1 digestive biscuit 1 piece of fruit	20	*Supper* coffee or tea with milk 1 slice of fruit loaf low fat diet margarine 1 glass of tomato juice

Figure 5.3.4
Different diets for different therapies

Diet features	Types I and II with insulin injections	Type II without medication, or oral medication only
energy intake required	when underweight, more energy; when overweight, restrict energy	when overweight, restrict energy
regularity of carbohydrate intake during the day	as regular as possible	preferably regular
importance of regular eating schedule	very important	preferable
importance of intake of extra energy when physical activity is increased	important	sometimes important

Study activity 3

a. A 68-year-old patient in a hospital medical ward has been a diabetic since the age of six. His diet is similar to the one in Figure 5.3.3 but because of an additional health problem he now finds it very difficult to eat bread. Plan appropriate meals for his breakfast and dinner using the exchange list in Appendix 2, ensuring that the carbohydrate content of the meals remains similar.

b. A 48-year-old woman, 170 cm (5ft 7in) tall and weighing 72.5 kg (11 st 6 lb), has had diabetes mellitus since she was a child and injects herself with insulin. It will be her birthday soon, and she has asked whether she can have something special to eat that evening. On normal evenings she has a piece of fruit, a cup of tea, a digestive biscuit and a glass of milk. What would you advise?

c. Give five examples of foods that diabetics can eat without restriction (i.e. low energy foods without carbohydrates).

6. Sugar and sweeteners in the diabetic diet

a. Can a diabetic eat any sugar?
In the past, sugar was considered to be 'poison' for someone with diabetes. Research has shown, however, that if sugar is blended into a meal it has the same effect on the level of glucose in the blood as, for example, macaroni or spaghetti. Diabetic diets are, therefore, increasingly allowed to contain sugar in this blended form (that is, in combination with fat, protein, or dietary fibre). This would include foods such as digestive biscuits, wholemeal bread sand-

wiches spread with ordinary jam, and ready-made desserts. Protein and fat reduce the rate of digestion so that the carbohydrates are broken down to glucose very slowly and, as a result, the glucose reaches the blood very gradually. The British Diabetic Association recommends 25g of sucrose per day to be incorporated into a diet (in baking or as preserves) that is low in fat and high in dietary fibre. Sugar in coffee or tea or sweetened lemonade are not recommended because sugar in this direct form is absorbed too quickly by the blood.

It is still best to restrict the intake of sugar, whether direct or blended, because it provides only 'empty' energy and therefore should be used only sparingly in any healthy diet. However, allowing sugar in blended form has some advantages for diabetics: it means that they can select appropriate foods for themselves from set menus or buffets at parties and other social functions without having to draw attention to their special dietary needs. Furthermore, it may save them from having to buy special diabetic foods which are expensive and may often be unpalatable. Being able to take sugar in blended form may also make it easier for diabetic patients to comply with their diets.

b. Sweeteners

There are two kinds of sweetener that can be used as substitutes for ordinary sugar: those which provide energy and those which are energy-free.

Energy-free sweeteners contain saccharin, aspartame or acesulfame K (Figures 5.3.5 and 5.3.6). Most of these sweeteners can be used in baking or cooking, although aspartame loses its sweetening power when heated to high temperatures. It can, however, be mixed with hot liquids as well as cold and still retain its sweetening effect.

Sorbitol is an example of a sweetener containing energy. It contains as much energy as ordinary sugar, and is therefore unsuitable for patients who are overweight. It can be used for cooking or baking, and it is widely used in special diabetic products including lemonade, chocolate, jam, cake, sweets, and desserts. Only 40 grams of sorbitol should be taken in any one day, because excessive amounts can cause diarrhoea. Special care is required in monitoring intake because some products contain sorbitol in large amounts and it is a wise precaution to examine the sorbitol content of the product as specified on the label.

Figure 5.3.5
Energy-free sweeteners

tablets	containing saccharin	Hermesetas
	containing saccharin and acesulfame K	Natrena
	containing aspartame	Canderel, Nutrasweet
	containing aspartame and acesulfame K	Hermesetas, Flix, New Taste, Sweetex Plus
liquid	containing saccharin	Natrena, Hermesetas, Sweetex
powder	containing aspartame	Canderel powder, Natrena, Nutrasweet
	containing saccharin and acesulfame K	Sweet 'n Low

Another energy-containing sweetener which can be used as a substitute for sugar is fructose or fruit sugar. Fructose has no side-effects, no bitter aftertaste, and it can be used in cooking or baking. However, unlike the rest of the sweeteners listed here, it contains carbohydrates and therefore cannot be used freely.

Study activity 4

A patient who has been prescribed the diet in Figure 5.3.3 would like to make some changes to it, and a fellow patient has told him that some sugar can be used in diabetic diets nowadays. He would like:
- a mug of cocoa with sugar instead of a glass of semi-skimmed milk in the morning
- a bowl of custard with sugar instead of a bowl of custard without sugar as a dessert
- a jam sandwich instead of a peanut butter sandwich in the evening.
  a. Do you think his wishes should be granted? Explain your answer.
  b. What would be the consequences of the changes to the diet?
  c. Work out how much additional carbohydrate he would ingest if these proposed changes were made to his diet.

Study activity 5

a. Name at least one advantage and one disadvantage for diabetics using energy-free sweeteners.
b. Sugar in blended form, such as in digestive biscuits, may be allowed in a diabetic diet. Does that mean that digestive biscuits can be eaten freely? Explain your answer.

7. Special diabetic foods

Products which are specifically intended for diabetics are always clearly labelled 'for diabetics', 'does not contain sugar' or 'suitable for diabetics'. In the future, however, these products may be labelled 'sweetened with ...', so that the diabetic can be sure that he or she is purchasing a product in which the sweetening agent is rich in 'empty' calories. There is little point in diabetics ingesting other energy-containing sweeteners as substitutes for sugar, since they are often overweight. In addition, ordinary products containing blended sugar (such as digestive biscuits, wholemeal bread, and ordinary jam) can be eaten by diabetics only in moderation, while there is a growing range of products aimed at the general consumer which contain artificial sweeteners.

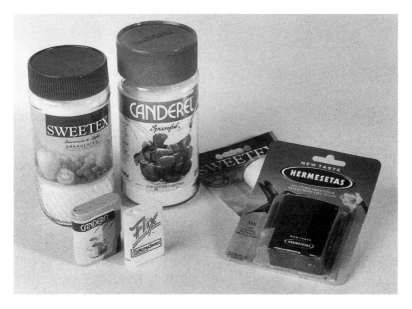

Figure 5.3.6
Sweeteners

The variety of special products available for diabetics includes jam, biscuits, ice-cream, confectionery, chewing-gum, lemonade, soft drinks and desserts. These products cannot, however, be consumed freely. They often contain great quantities of fat, protein, or carbohydrates and they may also contain sorbitol. Products like these must, therefore, replace part of the normal diet and not be taken in addition to it. Consequently, medical opinion suggests that 'normal' foods should be used in preference.

Study activity 6

a. What are the merits and disadvantages of using special low sugar diabetic products? When do you think it would be appropriate to use them?
b. Mrs Brown is 40 years old and has had diabetes for two years now. She uses sweeteners in her drinks and puts at least two in each cup of tea or coffee. What is your opinion about this? Explain.

Figure 5.3.7
Alcohol with snacks

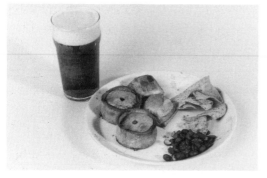

8. Alcoholic drinks and diabetes mellitus

In general, diabetics may drink a limited amount of alcohol and one or two drinks a day should not adversely affect the regulation of glucose in the blood. Alcohol lowers the level of glucose in the blood, and it is therefore best to drink alcohol only with a meal, or with a snack containing carbohydrates (Figure 5.3.7).

The energy content of alcohol makes it less suitable for diabetics who are overweight, and drinks containing carbohydrates (such as sweet wine, cream sherry and liqueurs) are not suitable for diabetics as they have a high sugar content. Thus, dry wines or spirits are preferred, together with low calorie tonics and lemonade or mineral/soda water.

Figure 5.3.8
Signs of hypoglycaemia and hyperglycaemia

Hypo	Hyper
Changeable temper	Drowsiness
Headache	Exhaustion
Exhaustion	Dry tongue
Pallor	Thirst
Hunger	Frequent urination
Sweating	
Tremor	
Impaired vision	
Dizziness	

Study activity 7

An 80-year-old man, 176 cm (5 ft 9 in) tall and weighing 73 kg (11 st 7 lb), has recently been diagnosed as diabetic. He takes an oral hypoglycaemic agent twice a day. He drinks three glasses of whisky every evening, and he asks whether he can continue. What advice would you give him, and why?

9. Special situations

a. Hypoglycaemia (level of glucose in the blood under 3 mmol/litre)
A sudden hypoglycaemia can develop when a diabetic patient has eaten too little or has left too long a gap between physical activity and eating. It can also be incited by injecting too much insulin, or by a very stressful situation. The symptoms are shown in Figure 5.3.8.

One of the following measures should cause these symptoms to disappear fairly rapidly:

– two or three lumps of sugar or fructose tablets, or
– a sweet drink, sweetened yoghurt, or yoghurt with rosehip syrup.

The diabetic should then eat one or two slices of bread, or some more yoghurt with fruit, or a few crackers, as sugar taken at the start of the hypoglycaemic attack will have been used up quickly and another 'hypo' might result.

b. Sports or physical activities

Regular exercise benefits our health in general, but it is particularly beneficial for diabetics, because a sedentary life reduces the effectiveness of insulin. There is no reason why diabetics should not participate in most sports as far as their abilities will allow (Figure 5.3.9).

Figure 5.3.9
Participation in sports

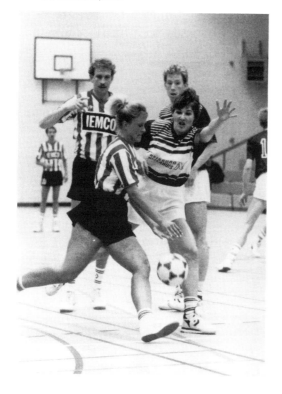

During sports or other strenuous physical activity, the body uses up more energy and thus more glucose. As a result, the food intake of diabetics who inject insulin must be adapted accordingly. The general recommendation is to eat an extra sandwich or its equivalent before physical activity, and to have a snack, if possible, during the activity. Physical activity reduces the need for insulin so that no extra injections are necessary.

c. Illness

When a diabetic is ill, and especially when he or she is running a temperature, more insulin than normal is needed. Treatment with insulin injections or with tablets which lower the level of glucose in the blood will have to be continued even if the diabetic is feverish and refuses to eat. It is not necessary to force the patient to eat, because diabetics rarely develop hypoglycaemia when they are ill, but it is very important for the patient to drink enough to prevent the dehydration which may result from the combination of fever and glucose loss in the urine.

A patient who feels sick, has appetite loss, but has no other symptoms of illness, must maintain his or her diet. The nursing staff must note whether a patient finds difficulty in eating, and they must notify the ward sister, the doctor and the dietitian when problems do occur so that the patient's diet and medication can be better adjusted to his or her needs.

d. Diabetes and pregnancy

If a diabetic woman plans to have a baby, it is very important that her blood glucose level be maintained between 4 and 7 mmol/litre before conception and during pregnancy. This can be done by the use of insulin and other means, and it will reduce the risk of congenital abnormalities, miscarriage, premature birth, and excessive birth weight.

Women who are not normally diabetic may become so during pregnancy if they are unable to produce the increasing amount of insulin that is required. This is called gestational diabetes, and the condition normally disappears when the insulin requirement normalises again after pregnancy. Strict regulation of the glucose level is achieved through diet, possibly in combination with insulin injections. Note that the diet will have to fulfil the special requirements of pregnancy, as described in Chapter 4 of Module 2.

e. The regulation of diabetes with the use of an insulin pump or an insulin injection pen
The insulin pump and the insulin injection pen are both devices which imitate the pancreas' natural production of insulin to attain precise regulation of the diabetes.

The insulin pump is carried on the body, and it contains a tiny motor which continually releases a small amount of insulin into the body. The natural production of extra insulin while a meal is being digested can be copied by pushing buttons on the pump to release an extra dose.

Unlike the pump, the insulin injection pen does not release insulin continuously. In the evening, a single dosage of long-term working insulin is injected. In addition, before each meal (up to three or four times a day) an extra quantity of short-term working insulin is injected from the insulin injection pen. The dose can be varied by pushing a button the appropriate number of times. The insulin injection pen is easy to use and unobtrusive.

These devices have the great advantage of giving users flexibility in the timing of their meals. The amount of insulin injected can be adjusted depending on the amount of carbohydrate taken, and it becomes much easier to cope with ordinary events such as holidays, parties, sporting activities or even a change in sleeping times at the weekend. It is essential, of course, that users regulate their own needs carefully.

10. Diabetes in children

From a very early age, diabetic children are expected to cope independently with their condition. Assisting and informing both parents and children is thus very important, and the information should always be made as accessible as possible to the children (through the use of cartoons, for example).

When there is a great deal of variation in physical activity or too much stress (possibly arising from problems at home or at school), deregulation of the diabetes can occur. During any periods when the child's glucose level is being regulated it is best to treat the child as an outpatient so that school attendance is not interrupted. However, it is not always possible to avoid hospitalisation, especially during periods when the child is growing rapidly.

When planning a diet, it is important to ensure that the child does not feel excluded from his or her peer group through its use at school, or from family activities in the home, and the special dietary requirements for optimal growth and development outlined in Chapter 4 of Module 2 should be a further important consideration.

Study activity 8

Jane is 15 years old and has been hospitalised with hyperglycaemia. The doctor has diagnosed diabetes mellitus. On admission, her glucose level was 27 mmol/litre. At first, she was given glucose, NaCl, and insulin intravenously, but now she is ready to start eating again. She is very thirsty, and drinks at least one litre of unsweetened apple juice and bitter lemon a day.

 a. Do you think her choice of drinks, and the quantity drunk, is appropriate during the regulation phase of diabetes mellitus?
 b. List some other beverages that you think would be suitable.
 c. After Jane had been on the ward for a few days and was progressing well, the dietitian gave her dietary advice and an extensive carbohydrate exchange list. The following weekend one of the ladies on the ward had a

birthday and treated everybody to apple pie. Jane's carbohydrate exchange list states that a slice of apple pie contains 26 grams of carbohydrate. Her dietary advice sheet states that during the afternoon she can have the following:

- 1 slice of brown bread with diet margarine, cheese or meat
- 1 piece of fruit
- 1 glass of semi-skimmed milk.

Jane asks you whether she can have the apple pie that afternoon. What would you advise?

Study activity 9

A 57-year-old man has recently been admitted to the medical ward of a hospital with cardiac problems. He has had diabetes mellitus since his youth. After a normal breakfast, during which he seemed in good spirits, he reported to physiotherapy for his treatment. Upon his return just before lunch time, he said he was very hungry. He was perspiring heavily, he looked pale and seemed exhausted. When questioned, his answers were rather incoherent.

  a. What may be wrong with this man?
  b. What would your response be?

Figure 5.3.10
© Nestlé Dietetic Information Services, U.K.

Myths about Diabetes

by Michael Cooper

Radical reforms in diabetic nutrition took place in the early 1980s, bringing the diet for people with diabetes into line with general recommendations for the whole nation. However, even now, myths about diabetes and food still exist.

SINCE THE DISCOVERY of insulin in 1922, the diabetic diet has undergone a complete metamorphosis. Dietary recommendations today – a high fibre. low fat diet – are the antithesis of the dietary recommendations of those early years. Then, a high fat, low carbohydrate diet was advised, with fat comprising 71% of the total calories. Radical reforms in diabetic nutrition took place in the early 1980s, bringing the diet for people with diabetes into line with the general recommendations for the whole nation. However, even now, myths about diabetes and food still exist. A few of the most persistent ones are listed below.:

Eating too much sugar and/or junk food causes diabetes.

Diabetes is not caused by anything you eat. However, eating lots of sweet and fatty foods may cause you to put on weight. Being overweight can increase the chance of developing non-insulin dependent diabetes, especially if there is a family history of this condition.

People with diabetes can't eat sugar.

Although it is important to restrict the amount of sugar and sweet foods you eat, it is neither practical nor necessary to avoid sugar altogether. Many foods contain sugar, even savoury foods such as bread, soups and baked beans. However, the amount of sugar in these foods is small and should not affect blood glucose levels. Home bakers can even include small amounts in their baking, providing it is included as part of a healthy diet, and they are not trying to lose weight.

If you have diabetes, you need special food.

You do not. Special diabetic foods are not necessary. They are expensive, they may contain a lot of fat, and, if eaten in large quantities, many have a laxative effect. It is far better to look for the low calorie, sugar-free and low fat foods which are readily available in most shops. These foods are suitable for anyone who wants to eat a healthier diet, and they are therefore useful for people who have diabetes.

People with diabetes can only eat small amounts of bread and potatoes.

Wrong. People with diabetes are encouraged to eat high fibre foods such as wholemeal bread. Jacket potatoes, brown rice, pasta, beans, oats and wholemeal breakfast cereal should make up the main part of the meal. High fibre foods are good for general health, but they can also help control the level of fat and sugar in the blood.

Having diabetes makes you fat.

Diabetes does not make you fat, and most people taking insulin are not overweight at all. However, the majority of diabetics controlled by tablets or diet alone need to lose weight, and this excess weight probably contributed to the development of diabetes in the first place. The British Diabetic Association works hard to dispel these myths and advises people on nutrition and all other aspects of living with diabetes. We are optimistic that over the next 10 years, myths associated with nutrition in the management of diabetes will start to fade away.

Study activity 10

An overweight man who suffers from maturity-onset diabetes is ill with a high temperature, and his appetite is severely depressed. What measures will have to be taken with regard to his diet?

11. Self-regulation

Nowadays, patients are encouraged to assume increasing responsibility for regulating their own diabetes. Self-regulation is the process whereby patients check their own blood and urine glucose levels, make their own decisions about their intake of food and assess their required dosage of insulin. Appropriate training, and support from the doctor, dietitian and nursing staff play a vital role in this. Patients have to learn to trust their own skills and abilities.

Self-regulation is especially useful when a person feels less fit or is under stress, on holidays, at parties, after exercise, or during menstruation. It is imperative that self-regulation be carefully carried out when the insulin pump or the insulin injection pen is being used.

12. Common misconceptions about diabetes

Figure 5.3.10 points out some of the more widespread myths about diabetes.

Study activity 11

At 7 o'clock in the evening, there is an acute admission of a 17-year-old patient with a blood glucose level of 28 mmol/litre. Diabetes mellitus is diagnosed, and insulin is administered slowly over a 24-hour cycle. The patient is concerned and upset, and he complains of being very thirsty. Since food is one of the highlights of his life, he repeatedly inquires about the future implications of his condition and its dietary restrictions.

a. As a nurse, what are the problems you would deal with?
b. In what order would you deal with them?
c. What would your aims be?
d. What actions would you have to take to achieve these aims?

13. Summary

Two forms of diabetes mellitus can be distinguished: insulin-dependent and non-insulin-dependent diabetes. Each type requires the treatment to be adapted to the individual's need. Therapy for a type I diabetic usually consists of a diet and insulin injections, while for type II diabetics a diet is often sufficient, though sometimes tablets or insulin injections are additionally necessary.

When the patient is also overweight, loss of weight is often the main aim of the diet, and there is a chance that medication may be reduced or stopped after a normal body weight has been attained. The diabetic diet is essentially a normal healthy diet with the additional proviso that regular intake of carbohydrates during the day should be maintained so as to avoid marked fluctuations in the blood glucose level.

As diabetics have a higher than average risk of developing cardiovascular disease, attention to the quantity and type of fat in the diet is an additional important consideration. By using exchange lists, substitutions can be made for meals or parts of meals whilst keeping the amount of carbohydrates the same.

There are a number of factors, such as physical activity, that can influence the level of glucose in the blood, and these have to be considered when assessing food intake or when calculating the required insulin dosage. The use of an insulin pump or an insulin injection pen gives greater flexibility in choosing the quantity of food eaten and the timing of meals, but it is essential for this use to be accompanied by adequate knowledge and careful self-regulation.

Diet and the pathology of the gastrointestinal tract

1. Introduction

Diet can play a significant role in disorders of the gastrointestinal tract. It is very common for patients with digestive tract complaints to have the feeling that meals are lying heavy in the stomach and to pinpoint specific foods as the ones which cause problems. Consequently, certain foods are promptly eliminated from the diet and, as symptoms worsen, there is danger that an ever-growing variety of foodstuffs will be avoided because of the fear of the pain, nausea, or diarrhoea that they are suspected of causing.

A huge variety of diets have been prescribed for gastrointestinal complaints over the years, and many of them (such as the special gastric diet, for example) are no longer regarded as useful. Most of the problems associated with specific foods depend upon the response of the individual, so it is often impossible to provide standard dietary advice for the various gastrointestinal disorders.

A few specific diets are given in this chapter, but for the most part a range of nutritional guidelines is all that can be offered.

Learning outcomes

After studying this chapter the student should be able to:
- explain briefly why special diets are often of minimal use in the treatment of disorders of the gastrointestinal tract;
- provide advice on how to alleviate the problems resulting from a hiatus hernia, and explain why this advice may be important;
- provide dietary advice to a patient suffering from a peptic ulcer;
- explain why someone whose stomach has been surgically reduced may drink nothing at all or only very little with their meals;
- distinguish between two forms of diarrhoea, and list a number of ways in which food can cause diarrhoea;
- list the most important points to be taken into consideration in cases of diarrhoea;
- list five drinks which can be given to patients with diarrhoea;
- state which foods may be eaten by patients suffering from coeliac disease or lactose intolerance;
- briefly describe the kinds of food which are suitable for patients with a colostomy;

- explain what is meant by constipation and state a possible long-term consequence of the condition;
- suggest four ways in which constipation can be caused by food;
- give six recommendations for the alleviation of constipation, and use these to plan a daily menu for a patient displaying signs of constipation;
- give two general considerations for treating patients with disorders of the gastrointestinal tract.

2. Diet and disorders of the oesophagus

a. Achalasia

Achalasia is a disorder of the lower oesophageal sphincter which normally allows food to pass to the stomach. Consequently, delay in the transit of food can occur and indigestion can become a serious problem. The patient often becomes afraid to eat and so loses weight. High energy fluids and finely chopped or easily digestible food should be given, normally in relatively small quantities.

b. Hiatus hernia and reflux oesophagitis

A hiatus hernia (Figure 5.4.1) is a protrusion of the stomach through the diaphragm. This means that the acidic contents of the stomach can easily pass upwards into the oesophagus, causing acid burning and occasionally reflux oesophagitis. In the acute stage, the drinking of milk may be encouraged in an attempt to buffer the effects of the gastric acids.

Hiatus hernia is a common problem of middle age, and it does not always lead to a more serious disorder. A hiatus hernia can result from being overweight, chronic coughing, or long-term constipation. There is also a congenital form.

The following advice will help to alleviate the symptoms of a hiatus hernia:
- Ensure that appropriate body weight is maintained;
- Eat small meals at regular intervals;
- Do not eat meals shortly before going to bed. It is advisable to eat the last meal of the day at least three hours before retiring to bed;
- Consume only a minimal amount of fat;
- Do not eat foods which can cause indigestion, such as onion, radish, red pepper, cucumber or fizzy drinks; orange juice and coffee may also cause problems;
- Do not drink alcohol;
- Ensure that bowel movements are regular;
- Do not wear tight-fitting clothes, and avoid bending and lifting;
- Do not lie down or sleep directly after a meal;
- Raise the head of the bed.

Figure 5.4.1
Different forms of hiatus hernia

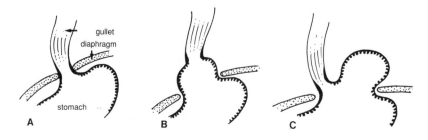

gullet
diaphragm
stomach
A   B   C

c. Obstruction

Disorders of the oesophagus may cause obstruction or blockage of the upper digestive tract. Such disorders include narrowing of the oesophagus (stenosis), or a tumour. A patient with an obstruction often becomes afraid to eat and may lose a considerable amount of weight. One possible solution is to give the food in liquid or finely chopped form (see Chapter 6 of this module). Encouraging the patient to sit upright while eating will assist the smooth passage of food, and artificial saliva may also assist swallowing.

d. Oesophageal varices

Oesophageal varices are often a complication of portal hypertension caused by cirrhosis of the liver. A special diet is not usually necessary, but hard bits in food such as fish or chicken bones and fruit pips, can cause bleeding of these varicose veins in the oesophagus, and these foods should therefore be avoided.

Study activity 1

Study the list of recommendations for alleviating the symptoms of a hiatus hernia, and explain in your own words how each recommendation works and why it is useful.

3. Diet and stomach complaints

a. Stomach ulcers

Until recently, a special diet was an important part of the treatment for a peptic ulcer. However, comparative research and practical experience have shown that the following guidelines are satisfactory to enable patients with gastric or duodenal ulcers to regulate their food intake:

- Eat food which is wholesome and rich in dietary fibre. It is not necessary to drink a lot of milk, but this can help to alleviate some of the symptoms;
- If specific foods are causing problems, avoid them for a while but try them again later;
- Eat slowly and chew well. Try to eat in a relaxed atmosphere, as tension can stimulate the stomach to produce more acid, which can aggravate the ulcer;
- Large meals are best avoided, as is eating shortly before going to bed, since eating late can cause problems during the night;
- There are a few items that should be avoided, such as fizzy drinks and alcohol. Coffee and tea with milk can be drunk if desired, but only during or immediately after a meal;
- Do not smoke. If you must smoke, do so only immediately after a meal. Smoking can irritate the mucous membrane in the stomach so if you do manage to stop, the ulcer will heal more rapidly.

In cases of peptic ulcers, there is enormous variation in the choice of food products that may be eaten, depending on the individual patient and on his or her reactions following consumption of the various foodstuffs. These personal experiences should be the prime consideration when planning the diet.

b. Gastric bleeding

Bleeding of the stomach usually occurs as a complication of peptic ulcers. Initially the patient will be given nothing orally, but a glucose-saline solution will be administered by drip. When the bleeding has stopped, the patient is started on a liquid diet or on food which is easily digested, and then gradually returned to a normal diet.

c. Stomach resection

A stomach resection in which part or all of the stomach is removed may be required in the case of a recurrent ulcer or in the case of cancer (Figure 5.4.2). One result of this is that the patient may sometimes suffer from dumping syndrome after meals. This occurs when the stomach is unable either to digest food properly or to store it adequately and results in large quantities of food being immediately passed (or 'dumped') into the intestine. The intestine then becomes distended, causing feelings of bloatedness, pain, nausea, dizziness, perspiration, and diarrhoea.

Dumping syndrome can be minimised or avoided by observing the following rules:
- Eat small meals frequently rather than large ones at long intervals;
- Drink little or nothing with meals so that the reduced stomach will be better able to digest the food;
- Ensure that the food is wholesome, and eat it slowly, chewing well;
- Sugar, products with high sugar content, and sweet dairy products can aggravate the condition and lead to symptoms of reactive hypoglycaemia. This is caused by the increased production of insulin in response to the high levels of glucose rapidly entering the bloodstream. Symptoms occur 1-2 hours after the meal and is known as late dumping syndrome.

Study activity 2

a. Why might someone who has had a stomach resection have to eat 6-10 times a day?
b. Why might eating a piece of fruit cake cause problems for someone who has had a stomach resection?

4. Diet and intestinal disorders

a. Diarrhoea

Diarrhoea is the most common disorder of the intestines. The symptoms are frequent, watery stools. Two forms of the condition, acute diarrhoea and chronic diarrhoea, can be distinguished.

Acute diarrhoea is generally severe in nature but brief in duration. It is usually the result of eating food or drinking water which is infected with bacteria or viruses (see Chapter 3 of Module 3), and it is, in fact, the body's normal response of attempting to expel these harmful infections or toxins from the body.

In addition, diarrhoea can be a symptom of a number of diseases, a result of anxiety or stress, or it may be precipitated by food containing too many carbohydrates (such as when children have eaten too many sweets and suffer an attack of diarrhoea some time later). If someone is accustomed to a diet with a low fat content, the sudden intake of excess fat can also trigger diarrhoea.

Chronic diarrhoea can occur when certain illnesses cause disorders of the digestive tract. Such ailments include lactose intolerance, coeliac disease, Crohn's disease, ulcerative colitis (all of which are covered later in this chapter), and diseases of the pancreas (covered in the next chapter).

Figure 5.4.2
Reduced stomach after a partial resection
(Billroth I anastomosis)

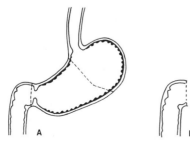
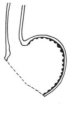
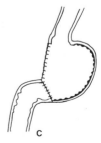

Patients suffering from diarrhoea, especially if it is severe, tend not to feel very hungry. It is extremely important, however, that they drink enough in order to prevent dehydration. In this respect, special attention must be paid to infants, toddlers, the elderly and patients who are weak.

Drinks suitable for patients with diarrhoea are water, fruit juices (such as apple juice, grape juice or blackcurrant juice), and tea; clear soup with no fat content can also compensate for salt lost as a consequence of diarrhoea. If diarrhoea continues, oral sodium chloride capsules can be administered.

When the diarrhoea subsides and the patient feels hungry again, carefully selected food can be given in small quantities. The cause of the diarrhoea will be a factor in deciding what can be eaten, but a few dry biscuits are often a good way to begin. It is still very important to drink enough, but fizzy drinks are not recommended.

As the appetite returns, the patient can usually eat anything he or she likes. Normally, initial choice will instinctively be small portions low in fat and dietary fibre. The resumption of a normal diet will be gradual and, in general, adults will not require any special dietary advice during this period.

Diarrhoea in children may have a variety of causes, ranging from the chronic forms to attacks brought on by incorrect bottle-feeding. In breast-fed infants, the cause may lie in the mother's diet. A child may also be hypersensitive to food (see Chapter 10 of this module). Dietary care will usually consist of a short period (usually 6 hours or more, but never more than 24 hours) when no food will be given though fluid will be administered parenterally, usually along with NaCl (for infants and toddlers). Normal food is then reintroduced gradually, beginning with heavily diluted food given in small quantities. After 5-10 days, depending on the course of the illness, the child should be able to revert to a normal diet.

In cases of acute diarrhoea in toddlers and pre-school children, no solid food should be given on the first day, but the loss of fluids and salt from the body necessitate an adequate fluid intake by the child. Suitable drinks include water, clear soup, tea (with glucose if desired), diluted fruit juice with glucose, and squash made from rosehip syrup. Large quantities of apple juice are not recommended.

When the diarrhoea subsides and the child wants to eat again, appropriate solid foods include dry biscuits or slightly stale white or light brown bread. A small serving of hot food can be tried. Failing any adverse reaction, the child can gradually resume a normal diet, but it is not recommended to start immediately serving meals high in fat content.

Study activity 3

Mrs Clarke, a 75-year-old widow, has been in hospital for a few weeks with injuries she sustained in a road accident. She has contracted an infection and is suffering increasingly from diarrhoea, with the result that she now refuses to eat or drink for fear that the diarrhoea will become more severe. She feels very weak, and blood tests have revealed anaemia.

    a. To which of Mrs Clarke's problems would you give priority attention?

    b. What aims should be set in the nursing of this patient? What should be done to achieve those aims?

    c. Would you advise that Mrs Clarke be given nothing to eat for a few days? Explain your answer.

b. Lactose intolerance

Lactose is a sugar in milk. When we drink milk or ingest milk products, the lactose component in the milk is broken down into glucose and galactose by an enzyme called lactase in our intestinal flora, so that it is in a state in which it can be absorbed into our bodies. However, some people have lactose intolerance, which means that the lactose they ingest cannot be broken down by lactase in their intestines into a state in which it can be absorbed. Instead, the lactose provides nutrients for gas-forming intestinal flora, so that when people suffering from the condition drink milk or ingest milk products, flatulence and abdominal cramps result, and sometimes diarrhoea in which the faeces have a watery, fermented consistency.

Lactose intolerance can be caused by:
- lactase deficiency, which may be
  - congenital;
  - primary lactase deficiency (in some non-Caucasian population groups, lactase activity drops to 10% after the first few years of life);
  - secondary lactase deficiency (in which some disorder of the gastrointestinal tract has, possibly temporarily, caused a lactase deficiency);
  - the ingestion of large quantities of lactose (even when there is sufficient lactase);
- a small bowel resection resulting in rapid transit of food through the shortened intestine, so that the lactose has not been broken down when it passes into the intestine, despite the presence of sufficient lactase in the stomach.

In most cases, a lactose-restricted diet is prescribed, which means that dairy products are largely or totally avoided. Lactose-free or lactose-reduced milks are available from supermarkets, however, and these may be tolerated. Commercial low lactose products may also be prescribed.

For those suffering from congenital lactase deficiency, a completely lactose-free diet is often necessary. All dairy products, and industrially prepared foods containing lactose (such as bread, biscuits, cakes, margarine, sausages, soups and sauces) must be avoided. Lists of lactose-free products are issued by the British Dietetic Association (see Appendix 3). Special lactose-free milk and soya milk, which is also lactose-free, can be used as substitutes for ordinary milk.

Deficiencies in calcium and vitamin B_2 may arise and, where this occurs, sup-

plements should be taken (though some brands of soya milk are available which contain added calcium and vitamin B_2, and these should prevent deficiencies). Special soya-based lactose-free food for babies and infants is also available.

Case study

Mrs Roberts, who is 63, began to experience difficulty swallowing her food. Even small mouthfuls posed a problem. Her doctor diagnosed a narrowing of the oesophagus, and advised her to take as much food as possible in the form of fluids, so she began to eat more porridge and desserts – things she had seldom eaten before.

At first, this worked well, but after a week she suffered from severe diarrhoea. Tests revealed that her body was unable to break down the increased amount of lactose she was ingesting, and a dietitian prescribed a lactose-restricted diet. From then on, her porridge and desserts were prepared with low lactose milk and, within a short time, the diarrhoea stopped.

c. Coeliac disease
In coeliac disease, the mucous membrane of the small intestine and the intestinal villi are damaged, leading to inadequate digestion and impaired resorption of nutrients in the small intestine. This often causes diarrhoea and undernourishment.

Coeliac disease is caused by a sensitivity to gluten, a protein which is found in wheat, rye, oats and barley. Gluten is therefore present in products like bread, biscuits and pastry. If a gluten-free diet is adhered to, the mucous membrane may heal, but the diet will have to be maintained for the rest of the patient's life. This will obviously have a significant impact on the patient (in some cases even small crumbs of bread can cause severe symptoms) and it is important to ensure that patients with poor nutritional status are given additional energy and nutrients in their diets. Temporary lactose intolerance can occur, necessitating a lactose-restricted diet.

Coeliac disease may also be accompanied by diarrhoea caused by excess fat in the diet, and when this happens a low fat diet is recommended.

In a gluten-free diet:

- ordinary bread must be replaced by bread made from wheat starch or special gluten-free flour. Such bread is often difficult to obtain and may therefore need to be home-baked;

- biscuits, pastry, pasta, binding agents, and industrially prepared products all have to be gluten-free. Purchases should therefore be checked against the list of commercially available gluten-free products which is published annually by the Coeliac Society (see Appendix 3), the association which offers information and advice to people with coeliac disease in the UK.

d. Colostomy and ileostomy

In cases of serious intestinal disease, such as Crohn's disease, ulcerative colitis, necrosis and tumours, it is sometimes necessary to surgically remove a section of the diseased intestine and fashion a new opening by which waste matter can leave the body. A colostomy is an artificial opening from the large intestine, and an ileostomy is an artificial opening from the small intestine (Figures 5.4.4 and 5.4.5). Stools are usually excreted into a bag which is sealed onto the opening.

Ileostomy often presents greater problems for the patient, as the entire large intestine has been removed, and the consequences include:

- frequent stools which are thin or fluffy;
- a tendency for excessive fat intake to trigger attacks of diarrhoea;
- irritation of the skin, if leakage occurs.

In addition, if there has been a resection of more than 70% of the small intestine (described as the 'short bowel

Figure 5.4.3a
Low lactose products

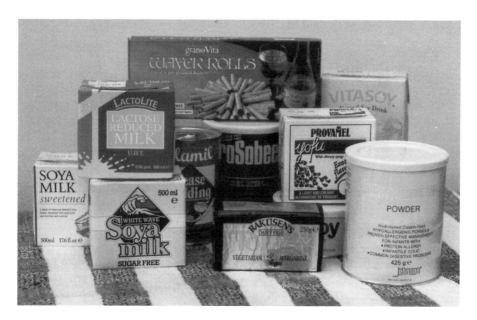

syndrome'), resorption of nutrients is insufficient so that vitamin and mineral supplements have to be taken. There is also a risk of lactose intolerance.

Following a colostomy, in which only part of the large intestine has been removed:

– stools tend to be infrequent although of normal consistency;
– there is a tendency to suffer from constipation;
– the skin is rarely irritated.

People with a colostomy or ileostomy do not require a special diet. They can determine for themselves what can and cannot be eaten. However, here are some general guidelines which will help to prevent the build-up of gases, unpleasant smells, and blockages of the artificial opening:

– Eating too quickly, talking whilst eating, and chewing gum will all lead to ingestion of air, thus increasing the volume of gas in the intestine. Some foods, in particular, create comparatively high volumes of gas in the body. These foods include pulses, new potatoes, fizzy drinks, beer, overcooked cabbage, Brussels sprouts, onions, garlic, leeks, mushrooms, milk, and sugar;
– Some strong-smelling foods, such as fish, onions, leeks, garlic, spices and eggs are not well tolerated;
– In cases of ileostomy, sufficient fluid intake is important, as is an adequate intake of salt, because much fluid and salt is eliminated with the stools;
– Some foods can cause blockages of the opening. Such foods include asparagus, apricots, nuts, citrus fruits, celery, mushrooms, and pulses. Chewing well or eating chopped or minced food can often prevent blockage;
– Blackcurrant juice, beetroot and spinach significantly affect the colour of the stools.

While patients can follow as normal a diet as possible, initially there may be considerable losses of both fluids and electrolytes in the stools. Diarrhoea may exacerbate these losses, and supplements of potassium (present in fruit juices) and sodium (present in sodium chloride supplements or salty foods) may be recommended.

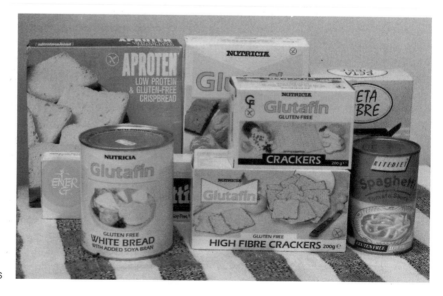

Figure 5.4.3b
Gluten-free products

Figure 5.4.4
Ileostomy

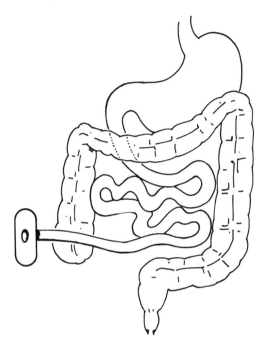

Figure 5.4.5
Colostomy

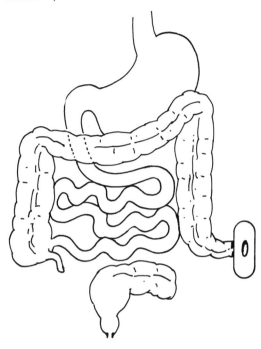

Study activity 4

Mr Sinclair, a 70-year-old bachelor, has been admitted to a nursing home to convalesce following intestinal surgery involving a colostomy. He used to work as a joiner and, since his retirement, he has enjoyed doing odd jobs for family and friends. However, around six months ago he began to suffer increasingly from abdominal pain and diarrhoea. Occasionally there were traces of blood in his stools. Cancer of the large intestine was diagnosed, and total excision of the carcinoma was effected about a month ago.

Mr Sinclair has been in the ward for a few days now, and he is still trying to adapt to the colostomy. He eats very little for fear of pain, especially avoiding vegetables and fruit, and he is convinced that everybody can see and smell his colostomy.

    a. How might you reduce Mr Sinclair's fear of pain and help him to become more accustomed to his colostomy?

    b. Do you think he should be advised against eating food which has a strong aroma or which causes flatulence?

The Ileostomy Association of Great Britain (see Appendix 3) is an association which offers help and advice to people who have undergone colostomies or ileostomies.

e. Constipation

Constipation literally means 'blockage' and, in practice, it means that a person defecates less often than is usual. Stools are harder and their quantity is reduced. Constipation may be accompanied by unpleasant side-effects such as headache, bloatedness, abdominal pain or loss of appetite. Long-term sufferers may develop haemorrhoids.

The most common causes of constipation are dietary in origin, and they include insufficient intake of dietary fibre and fluids, and eating too little or too irregularly. Ignoring the urge to defecate because of a rushed or irregular lifestyle can lead to constipation, because stools which stay in the body longer may become dry and difficult to pass. Lack of exercise, particularly amongst the elderly or bedridden, is another cause – 20% of people over

70 regularly suffer from the symptoms associated with constipation.

Other causes include disturbance of bowel function, diverticulosis, and the use of certain types of medication, including iron pills (prescribed for anaemia), antihypertensives, painkillers (especially potent drugs like morphine), and anti-depressants. The long-term use of laxatives may also suppress the natural movements of the intestine.

Study activity 5

a. Why do elderly people, patients in hospital and pregnant women often suffer from the symptoms associated with constipation?
b. The treatment of constipation is based on the increased amounts of dietary fibre in combination with an increased programme of exercise. Name six kinds of food that are rich in dietary fibre and state to which group of foodstuffs they belong.

Study activity 6

Mrs Foley is a 76-year-old widow with two daughters. A district nurse calls twice a week to care for her because she is deteriorating physically and beginning to show signs of dementia. Her daughters look after her the rest of the time. Mrs Foley has always been active, keen on knitting, playing cards, gardening and going for walks, but she now tends to spend most of her time indoors. She has become rather passive, watching TV all the time, and she says that she doesn't feel as well as she used to. She complains of headaches and a bloated feeling, and she also suffers from constipation.

Her daily meals are typically as follows:
Breakfast
- 2 slices of buttered toast (white bread) with marmalade
- 1 cup of tea
Lunch
- 1 cup of soup
- 2 potatoes

- 1 serving of vegetables
- 1 portion of meat and gravy
- 1 bowl of dessert or custard
Dinner
- 3 slices of white bread and butter, with cheese, ham or jam
- 1 cup of tea
Snacks
- 2 cups of coffee
- 2 cups of tea
- 2 biscuits
- 1 glass of milk
  a. What are the most likely causes of Mrs Foley's constipation?
  b. What should the nurse's aims be in this situation?
  c. How might these aims be achieved?

Sufficient intake of liquid when suffering from constipation is very important. It will assist the evacuation of faeces by allowing dietary fibre to absorb fluid, swell up, and stimulate bowel movement.
Guidelines for dealing with constipation
- Make sure that the diet is high in dietary fibre;
- Eat regularly and do not skip meals;
- Drink at least 1.5 litres of fluid a day;
- If you feel your bowels move, do not delay in going to the toilet, try not to suppress the urge;
- Try to go to the toilet regularly to encourage regular bowel movements, and take your time;
- If possible, take plenty of exercise;
- Avoid the use of laxatives (unless prescribed by a doctor).

Study activity 7

a. What is the connection between fluids and dietary fibre?
b. How can you tell whether a patient who appears to be constipated has been taking enough fluids?

High fibre foods
The following foods are rich in dietary fibre (see Figure 5.4.6):
- wholemeal foods, such as wholemeal

bread, wholewheat biscuits, muesli, oatmeal porridge, brown rice, and wholewheat pasta;
– pulses;
– fresh fruit, and dried fruit such as prunes, apricots, figs, currants, and raisins;
– vegetables, whether cooked or in a salad;
– beans (including baked beans), processed peas;
– nuts, peanut butter and sunflower, pumpkin, and sesame seeds.
Foods which contain a negligible amount of dietary fibre but which, nevertheless, have a laxative effect include:
– sour dairy products (e.g. yoghurt);
– orange juice and rosehip syrup.

Figure 5.4.6
Food rich in dietary fibre

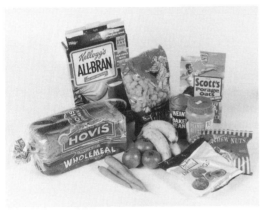

Some people suffering from constipation occasionally pass thin, watery stools. This is not diarrhoea but a side-effect of constipation sometimes called 'pseudo-diarrhoea' (or false diarrhoea). These cases also, therefore, will respond to a high fibre diet.

Study activity 8

Look again at Study Activity 6 and change Mrs Foley's daily menu to a high fibre dietary regimen. Take her total intake of fluids into account.

If the guidelines given above do not achieve the desired effect, the use of bran can be considered. Bran can cause flatulence and a feeling of bloatedness at first, however, so it is important to start with only three tablespoonfuls of bran a day, increasing this gradually to six. The bran can be mixed with yoghurt, custard, porridge, soup, stew, or vegetables. It can also be added to the fillings of sandwiches (with butter or margarine, peanut butter, or cream cheese) or taken with some water. The laxative effect of bran is greatest when taken regularly throughout the day, and when taken in conjunction with plenty of fluid.

The effect of bran is not always immediate and may not be noticeable for the first week or two.

f. Irritable bowel syndrome
Irritable bowel syndrome is a complex disorder which affects 10-35% of the population. Irritation of the intestine causes a range of symptoms, which may be constant or intermittent, and which have no obvious underlying cause. The activity of the entire gastrointestinal tract may be disturbed, and the symptoms vary widely and may include:
– diarrhoea or constipation or both;
– excessive gas formation;
– the elimination of fluids with the faeces;
– swelling of the abdomen.
Psychological problems can aggravate the problem. IBS tends to affect 'highly-strung', tense people where nerves supplying the bowel are overly excited.

Patients with irritable bowel syndrome are advised to follow a high fibre diet (even when diarrhoea is present), take plenty of fluids and eat at regular intervals. (See the guidelines given above for dealing with constipation.)

g. Diverticulosis and diverticulitis
When the wall of the large intestine becomes more distended than usual, this condition is described as diverticulosis.

Inflammation of the distended areas is known as diverticulitis. These disorders are very common, with about 35% of people over the age of 60 suffering from diverticulosis. One of the causes is thought to be the lack of dietary fibre in our Western diet (see Chapter 1 of Module 3).

A high fibre diet has a positive effect on the condition because it improves the bowel function and may minimise or even eliminate the associated symptoms.

h. Inflammatory diseases of the intestine
This category includes Crohn's disease and ulcerative colitis, both of which are characterised by chronic inflammation with alternating periods of remission and relapse.

Crohn's disease is usually localised in the terminal portion of the ileum and in the colon. Patients with Crohn's disease do not usually require specific dietary advice unless the condition is complicated by serious stenosis or the formation of a fistula. In those cases, parenteral feeding or liquid feeding (by tube if necessary) is undertaken. If surgery is required, an ileostomy may be created. A lactose-restricted diet is necessary in cases of lactose intolerance, and a low fat diet should be used where there is diarrhoea linked to excessive intake of fat.

As patients suffering from Crohn's disease often have poor nutritional status, the frequent serving of small meals high in energy and protein is recommended, particularly where the patients complain of loss of appetite. Additional fluids and minerals will be needed in the diet to compensate for any fluid loss which may occur as a result of diarrhoea.

Ulcerative colitis is usually localised in the colon (especially the rectum) although the small intestine can also be affected. In most cases blood and mucus are mixed with the stool, which is often thin and watery, and this may result in anaemia due to the lack of iron. Giving the patient additional iron can prevent or minimise the anaemia. In the acute stage, parenteral

or liquid feeding can be used. If the patient recovers, no special diet is necessary but, if lactose-intolerance is shown, a lactose restricted diet should be adhered to.

In both Crohn's disease and ulcerative colitis, the dietary measures taken will depend on the patient's individual symptoms. When the patient has no particular problems and is well nourished, the best recommendation is a nutritional and well-balanced diet following the general rules given earlier.

5. Providing guidance for patients with gastroenteric disorders

It can sometimes be difficult to deal with the dietary problems of patients who, by the nature of their illness, do not have much interest in food. Appetite tends to decrease as symptoms worsen, and if the patient avoids an ever-increasing variety of foodstuffs, the dietary variation becomes increasingly limited.

If special dietary advice is required at this time, it is usually only a temporary need. The most important task may be to direct the patient from a lifetime of unhealthy eating habits. Although it is not easy to change a patient's dietary pattern, there will be positive benefits for the patient's health if he is encouraged to gradually adopt as normal a diet as possible, and it is important to let patients discover for themselves the range of foods which they can eat and enjoy.

In the case of diseases where specific diets (such as gluten-free, lactose-free, or high in dietary fibre) may be required, there are a number of local and national associations and support groups which offer help and advice. The addresses of many of these organisations are listed in Appendix 3.

Study activity 9

Draw a sketch of the gastrointestinal tract. Identify the major structures mentioned in this chapter and label the diseases affecting these structures. Relate the diseases to the shape and function of the structures. Briefly identify principal dietary modifications that may be recommended for each disease.

6. Summary

Diet can play an important role in the treatment and control of gastroenteric problems. People who have such problems tend to restrict their diet unnecessarily.

Dietary guidelines have been given for disorders of the oesophagus, the stomach and the intestine. For most conditions, special dietary advice is only usually required for a short duration because often the patients themselves are best able to determine what to eat and what to avoid.

However, there are a number of gastroenteric complaints for which long-term diets are recommended.

Diet and the pathology of the liver, gall bladder, and pancreas

1. Introduction

Over the years, various diets have been prescribed for conditions of the liver, gall bladder, and pancreas, and much ill-founded and outdated advice is still being followed. However, the most appropriate diet for patients with these conditions is one matched to the individual preferences and symptoms of the patient. As in the case of gastroenteric conditions, strict diets are seldom necessary and the patient is more likely to benefit from sound, general dietary advice.

Learning outcomes

After studying this chapter the student should be able to:
- list a number of general points of advice for patients suffering from hepatitis, cirrhosis of the liver, or hepatic coma;
- list a number of dietary guidelines for patients with colic caused by gallstones;
- give two recommendations for the prevention of gallstones;
- give a number of examples of low fat foods suitable for patients with chronic inflammation of the pancreas.

2. Diet and the pathology of the liver

The liver (Figure 5.5.1) produces bile, which is needed for digestion, and it plays an important role in breaking down fats, proteins, carbohydrates, and alcohol in our bodies. It also neutralises degradation products and toxic substances. It is an extremely important and totally indispensable organ.

The most significant diseases of the liver are hepatitis, cirrhosis of the liver, and hepatic coma, and all of these disorders can severely affect liver function. In all cases, the appropriate diet will depend to a great extent on the severity of the condition.

a. Hepatitis

Hepatitis can be caused by a viral infection or by excessive use of alcohol. Special diets are not an integral part of treatment, but a healthy diet with a moderately restricted intake of fat is recommended. Given that the average Western diet has a high fat content, for many patients a lower fat diet is the chief recommendation in this respect.

Patients with hepatitis are likely to have a depressed appetite, and their preferences and symptoms should be taken into account as far as possible. Some patients, for example, are unable to digest fried foods very well, and smaller meals, served more frequently during the day, are often easier to digest than two or three large meals.

The diet of a patient with hepatitis should contain plenty of energy, since undernourishment will impair the liver's capacity to heal. Where the patient is very emaciated, parenteral feeding is often necessary. Alcohol is strictly forbidden, because of its effect on the liver.

Study activity 1

Patients with hepatitis should follow a diet containing only a moderate amount of fat. Make a list of foods suitable for inclusion in such a diet.

b. Cirrhosis of the liver

Cirrhosis of the liver is a chronic disease affecting the tissue of the liver. The main causes are long-term alcohol abuse, chronic infection and chronic obstruction of the gall-bladder.

In the early stages of the disease, the counselling given is identical to that given to hepatitis patients, and small, frequent meals are recommended. However, fluid and salt retention may occur in the form of ascites and oedema and, if this happens, a low sodium, low fluid diet is recommended. The diet must also be high in energy and protein to restrict the development of ascites.

c. Hepatic coma

When a disease such as hepatitis or cirrhosis prevents the liver from functioning, the liver becomes incapable of performing its usual role of detoxifying the degradation products of proteins. The resultant build-up of toxins can cause hepatic coma.

In the acute phase, nutrition is given parenterally, and will contain mainly carbohydrates and fat. This is followed by a low protein, high energy diet containing vitamins and minerals, and it may be necessary to alter the consistency of the diet at this stage to facilitate swallowing. As the patient's condition improves, the protein content of the food can be increased. Small and frequent meals are recommended as patients are likely to have depressed appetites.

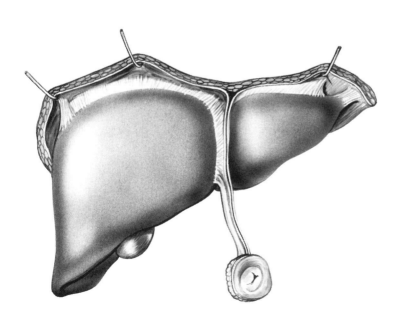

Figure 5.5.1
The liver

3. Diet and the pathology of the gall bladder and bile duct

a. Gallstones

Gallstones are one of the most common conditions of the bile duct, affecting about 15% of the population (rising to around 30% of those over 65 years old), and the incidence of the condition trebles amongst those who are overweight. Normally, people with gallstones are unaware of their condition. Only a small number suffer any symptoms. However, if one of the gallstones escapes from the gall bladder, and travels along the bile duct causing a blockage of the duct, this will result in severe pain known as colic (or biliary colic).

If a patient suffers from attacks of colic it is important to establish exactly which foods exacerbate the pain. Often it is meals with a high fat content and substances such as coffee, egg yolk, spinach, rhubarb, chocolate, cocoa and alcohol which cause the greatest problems, and it is obviously advisable to limit or avoid any foods which aggravate symptoms. Precisely which foods can be eaten will therefore depend on the individual patient.

If a patient with gallstones is free from symptoms, no special diet is required. However, to prevent gallstones, a healthy, high fibre diet is recommended. It may also be a preventative measure to eat later in the evening or have a snack just before bedtime. This will minimise the build-up of bile which occurs naturally overnight and which may subsequently promote gallstone formation.

b. After a gall bladder operation

No special diet is required after either laparoscopic investigation of the gall bladder or after its complete removal. The patient should gradually revert to a normal, healthy diet. In practice, a number of patients adhere to a stringent diet for the rest of their lives, and counselling should be offered to prevent them from limiting their diets unnecessarily and thus risking nutritional deficiencies.

Study activity 2

Is it advisable for a patient who has undergone gall bladder surgery three months ago to have a cup of coffee?

4. Diet and the pathology of the pancreas

When the pancreas (Figure 5.5.3) is diseased by chronic pancreatitis, cystic fibrosis or pancreatic carcinoma for example, its functions may be affected. Digestion may thus be impaired, and diabetes can occasionally develop. Insufficient digestion of fats can also lead to steatorrhoea (excess fat in the faeces which

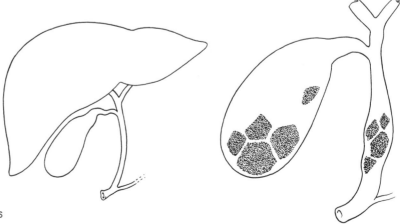

Figure 5.5.2
Gall bladder and gallstones

may cause diarrhoea) but taking pancreatic enzymes with meals can improve the digestion of fats. Reducing the amount of fat in the diet can help to alleviate the diarrhoea but over a long term a low fat diet may result in a deficiency of the fat-soluble vitamins (vitamins A, D, E and K). If the steatorrhoea persists, MCT (Medium Chain Triglycerides) are occasionally used in cases of extreme emergency. These are short chains of fatty acids which are directly absorbed into the intestine. Examples of MCT dietary products include Medium Chain Triglyceride Oil from Cow and Gate Nutricia, and Liquigen from Scientific Hospital Supplies.

Figure 5.5.3
The pancreas

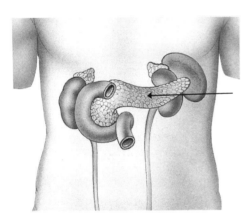

Small, frequent meals are also recommended for patients suffering from pancreatic disorders, since the pancreatic digestive juices are more capable of managing smaller quantities of food, and this can also help to relieve the pain. The patient is strongly encouraged to avoid alcohol, and high energy, high protein supplements for the diet may be used if the patient is emaciated or undernourished.

Study activity 3

a. Suggest a number of low fat meals which would be suitable for a patient with chronic pancreatitis.
b. Why do patients with disorders of the pancreas occasionally develop diabetes?

5. Summary

The most appropriate diet for a patient with a disorder of the liver, gall bladder, or pancreas is one adapted to the individual patient's preferences and symptoms. The avoidance of alcohol is highly recommended, but a stringent diet is seldom necessary and the patient is more likely to benefit from sound general dietary advice.

Food with an altered consistency

1. Introduction

Most of us are totally unaware of the fact that eating and drinking are extremely complex activities. Chewing and swallowing involve several muscle groups and nerves from the head and neck area. When a patient is unable to chew or swallow normally for psychological or physiological reasons, or when food is difficult to swallow, consumption of special foods may be necessary. Nowadays there are a number of options available for prescribing a fluid or liquidised diet, so that undernutrition can be prevented.

Learning outcomes

After studying this chapter the student should be able to:
- explain what is meant by 'food with an altered consistency', i.e. tube feed, monomeric, and polymeric feeds;
- briefly describe five situations in which food with an altered consistency may be necessary;
- describe a hot and cold meal which can be included in a soft diet;
- name one advantage and one disadvantage of maintaining a diet of soft or liquid food;
- provide a number of general dietary guidelines for irritations of the mouth or throat, the formation of mucus in the mouth and swallowing conditions;
- explain why foodstuffs such as cream, syrup, honey, sugar, glucose, dextrin-maltose, or a protein preparation are often added to a drink or to porridge in a liquid diet;
- give three reasons why it may be necessary to use a tube feed;
- give four important guidelines for administering tube feeds;
- indicate what important information should be given to a patient being administered tube feeds or monomerous feeding for the first time.

2. Examples of when food with an altered consistency is prescribed

Food with an altered consistency does not have the same solid texture as normal food. The food can be in fluid or liquidised form and is indicated for different reasons as follows:

- when there are problems chewing. This can occur when the mucous membrane of the mouth is inflamed, following extraction of a tooth or jaw operation, when dentures do not fit properly, following radiation treatment to the head or neck area, in hemiplegics or with AIDS patients;
- when there are problems swallowing. This can occur as a result of hemiplegia, spasticity, multiple sclerosis, Parkinson's disease, motor neurone disease, tumours in the pharynx, following a tonsillectomy, radiation therapy, and following a cerebrovascular accident (stroke);
- when there is inflammation or constriction of the oesophagus or the remainder of the gastrointestinal tract;
- when the patient is seriously fatigued;
- when there is an extreme loss of appetite;
- following extensive surgery;
- after protracted periods following digestive or absorption disorders.

The most appropriate consistency may be negotiated with the patient or following assessment, usually depending on the severity of the disorder.

3. Liquidised/minced food

In the examples in the previous subsection, eating bread, meat, pieces of fruit, and hard pieces of vegetables in particular may lead to problems. Sometimes it is sufficient to chop the food finely. The food then looks more appetising than it does when it is liquidised. In most cases, a liquidised diet may be given if finely chopped food still causes problems. Food such as meat and vegetables can be blended in a food processor.

Case study

Mr Baldwin is a 79-year-old man who had chewing problems because of his ill-fitting dentures. He has inflammation of the mouth, and cannot wear his dentures at the moment. After consultation between staff and patient, a liquidised/soft diet is chosen. His daily menu is as follows:

Breakfast
- scrambled egg
- 3 slices of brown bread, no crust, with butter, marmalade or jam
- 1 glass of milk
- cup of tea

Mid-morning snack
- white coffee
- soft roll or scone with butter
- soft fruit (bananas or sliced tinned peaches) or fresh fruit juice

Lunch
- bowl of soup
- portion of minced meat, chicken or fish
- portion of mashed potatoes
- portion of puréed or mashed vegetables such as cauliflower, carrots, or spinach
- bowl of chocolate pudding

Tea
- cup of tea with some softened biscuits
- fruit yoghurt

Dinner
- as breakfast

Supper
- cup of tea with milk
- soft roll with butter and cream cheese
- glass of fruit juice

Before bed
- glass of hot milk

Study activity 1

a. What are the advantages and the disadvantages of maintaining a diet of liquidised food?
b. If Mr Baldwin is unable to eat fresh fruit or drink fruit juice because of the inflammation in his mouth, how could

you make sure he receives sufficient vitamin C?

c. Why do you think that brown or wholemeal bread would be preferable to white bread in this situation? Are rusks likely to cause problems for Mr Baldwin?

4. Caring for patients on a liquid/soft diet

The practical care of patients on a liquid or soft diet demands special attention. It is especially important when there are long-term problems with chewing or swallowing to make sure that the menu does not become too limited and patients do not live on just milk desserts and porridge. If a well-balanced diet of liquidised/soft food (such as the case study sample diet) is prescribed promptly, undernutrition can be avoided.

Attention must also be given to the manner in which food is served. Food which has been liquidised or puréed is often unrecognisable. Telling the patient what the diet consists of may make the meal more appetizing. If the meat, vegetables and potatoes are kept separate they will be more easily recognisable and be more readily accepted. Taking the tastes and preferences of the patient into account is just as important in the case of liquidised food. Ensuring that the dishes are varied in colour, aroma and taste can prevent monotony.

5. Feeding liquidised food by tube

If a liquidised diet still causes problems, other alternatives are available. We can identify two kinds:

a. Home-made liquid food
Examples of food which may be used in a liquid diet:
Breakfast
porridge, tea, milk, yoghurt, fruit juice
Lunch
broth, smooth creamed soup, minced beef, shepherd's pie, fish, puréed vegetables;

mashed potatoes, fruit mixture (of puréed fruit), custard, yoghurt
Evening meal
broth, smooth creamed soup, porridge, custard, tea, coffee, milk, yoghurt
Snacks
coffee, tea, milk, milk shakes, yoghurt, finely minced fruit, fruit juice, cottage cheese, lemonade, vegetable juice. Proprietary drinks or desserts that are high in energy can be taken if necessary.

Guidelines for a liquid diet
– To increase the amount of energy in the food, the following can be added as needed: single cream, syrup, honey, glucose, dextrin-maltose, or other carbohydrate preparations (Figure 5.6.1);
– Sometimes, extra protein needs to be added. This could be a protein-rich preparation in powdered form and can be added to milk or soups;
– When a patient suffers from severe mouth irritation, blackberry juice can ameliorate the complaints. Very sour, salty, or sweet products, and strong spices make the symptoms worse. Sour food is easier to digest if cream is added;
– If a patient complains of mucus in the mouth, rinsing with fizzy mineral water, camomile tea and pineapple juice can help. The production of thin, watery saliva can be stimulated by chewing and by sour flavours. Products which are suitable for this are chewing-gum and boiled sweets;
– In the case of swallowing problems it is recommended to serve food that is concentrated and not too thin. Thick or thickened liquids such as yoghurt, porridge, custard and stews make swallowing easier, and reduce the risk of liquids getting into the lungs and causing discomfort;
– Make sure that plates and bowls are suitable for the type of food served and that they are hygienically and attractively presented;
– Make sure that the tastes of the foods are varied. For example, sweet and

savoury, sweet and sour, hot and cold. Colour variation is also important;
- Food should contain sufficient dietary fibre;
- Artificial saliva may be used to lubricate foods.

Study activity 2

a. Create a one-day menu for a patient with dysphagia secondary to motor neurone disease. He currently weighs 54.5 kg (8 st 8 lb) and he is 168 cm (5 ft 6 in) tall. Swallowing is very difficult for him so he requires a diet which is also high in energy. Pay attention to variation in flavours.
b. How do you know if this patient obtains sufficient fluid every day?

An important element of care for patients who are on a liquid diet is that fluid intake is being maintained. The risk of dehydration exists particularly with patients who have swallowing problems.

Recipe for an orange drink .
Mix the following ingredients: juice of one orange, one tablespoon of lemon juice, a mashed banana or three tablespoons of fruit purée, and three tablespoons of cream.

b. Proprietary Feeds
- Polymerous liquids
  These are liquids that contain normal, long chain fats, protein and carbohydrates. The patient digests and absorbs normally. Examples of situations in which polymerous liquids are given are found above in Section 2 of this chapter.
  Polymerous feeds are available in the following forms:
  - protein-enriched supplementary feeds in a variety of flavours;
  - sip feeds in different flavours;
  - tube feeds - these can also be used as sip feeds although the flavour may not be very palatable. To improve the flavour, instant coffee, cocoa powder, or rosehip syrup can be added.

- Monomerous liquids
  These are feeds in which protein, fat, and carbohydrate are pre-digested. The chain length of these macronutrients is short and therefore easy to digest and these are used when the digestive system and capacity to absorb food is reduced. The elemental nature of the feed means that it is quite concentrated. The flavour of the food is generally regarded as poor, although several flavours are available. This feed leaves little residue and is almost fully absorbed. This type of feed is given in the case of very severe digestive and/or resorption disorders, such as Crohn's disease, pancreatitis, or after surgery of the gastrointestinal tract.
  Some important guidelines for the care of patients on monomerous liquid feeds are:
  - the patient (and visitors) must be highly motivated and well instructed. The patient may, for instance, worry about the small quantity of stools produced;
  - the food should be at the correct temperature;
  - encourage the patient to drink slowly, so that feeling bloated, vomiting, and diarrhoea are prevented;
  - in most cases, tea, water, and clear soup may also be added to the diet;
  - additional clear fluids are encouraged to prevent dehydration;
  - a patient who has been on this kind of diet for a prolonged period may be given chewing-gum (if the disorder allows it), which has a positive effect on the chewing function.

Case study

Mrs Brooks is a 70-year-old widow with two children. Since her husband's death, she has been living with her eldest son. She suffered a cerebrovascular accident and was hospitalised. On examination, a hemiplegia on the right side was diagnosed. She now has problems speaking and swallowing.

When initially admitted to hospital, she was put on a tube feed which was later followed by a liquid diet. After five weeks in hospital, she indicated that she would prefer to go back to her son's home where she would be cared for by her family and the community nurse. Two months later, Mrs Brooks was hospitalised again because she had dehydration and acute loss of weight. When her family was contacted, the cause soon became clear: because of her swallowing problems, the patient had refused to eat anything except small quantities of porridge and custard. She drank very little because swallowing was painful.

Figure 5.6.1
Table of commercially prepared liquid foods

i. Polymerous liquids
- protein-enriched supplementary foods: Fortimel, Fortisip;
- complete drinking food*;
- tube feed*: Enrich, Ensure, Survimed, Pulmocare;
- feeds for children: Pediasure.

ii. Monomerous liquids
- complete drinking food*: Flexical, Pepti-2000;
- infants and children: Pepti-Junior.

*All these foods are complete and can also be administered by drip feed or through fistula.

Study activity 3

a. Name three conditions that would encourage the use of polymerous liquid feeds.
b. What do you think is important to tell a patient who is receiving monomerous sip feeds for the first time?
c. Name three conditions that indicate the use of monomerous sip feeds.

Figure 5.6.2

Examples of supplements containing carbohydrates:

Hycal	Polycal	Maxijul
Nutrical	Polycose	Fortical
Caloreen	Fortijuice	

Examples of supplements containing mainly proteins:

Protifar	Casilan	Maxipro
Vipro	Promod	Fresubin
Provide	Formance	Ensure
Build-Up	Fortisip	Entera
Forceval		

6. Tube feed

A tube feed is a complete liquid diet containing sufficient energy and nutrient, and which can be administered by means of a tube inserted through the mouth or nose, or through a surgically made opening in the abdominal wall (fistula) via gastrostomy or jejunostomy.

Tube feeds are administered to patients who are unable to take normal or liquid food orally, such as patients who are suffering from serious swallowing problems, who are unconscious, or have undergone extensive surgery to the head and neck area. Tube feeds are also administered when patients are too weak to eat or when patients do not want to eat while in a life-threatening situation, as can be the case with anorexia nervosa or serious depression.

a. Examples of tube feeds
- Proprietary feed (liquid or in powdered form)
  Liquid feeds are easy to use, hygienic, and available in a variety of types, e.g. high energy, high protein, low protein, low fat, fibre-enriched, lactose-free, low carbohydrate, soya protein-based. They can be kept at room temperature if left unopened.
  Tube feed in powdered form is usually soluble in water (follow instructions).

Hygiene is very important here because drip feed is an ideal breeding ground for bacteria. Insufficient hygiene can, for example, cause diarrhoea.

– Home-prepared tube feed
  Foodstuffs such as milk, meat, vegetables, potatoes, cream, fruit, and oil can be liquidised, thinned with milk or stock, and strained. The advantage of home-made tube feed is that it can be adapted to fit the individual patient's needs and can therefore meet special dietary demands. However, the extensive range of ready-made tube feeds available makes home preparation more and more unnecessary and, in most cases, inferior.

b. Guidelines for the use of tube feed
– Tube feed is administered either by drip or in small quantities at regular intervals during the day (and night if needed). Feeds must not be administered too quickly as the patient may experience an unpleasant, full feeling in the stomach, possibly leading to diarrhoea. When necessary, a 'starter' tube feed can be given. This is like a thinned tube feed but containing all the necessary nutrients;
– Bring the feed to room temperature. Feeds that are too cold can cause diarrhoea, vomiting, or a bloated feeling;
– Orange juice (vitamin C) cannot be given together with tube feed as the feed may curdle; it can be given after the tube feed;
– Rinse the tube and the dispensing system after each feed with 30-50 ml of water so that the drip does not become blocked;
– Do not use the tube feed longer than is indicated on the package. Opened bottles can be kept in the refrigerator for two days. Extra attention to hygiene is important when making a drip feed. Keep it for a maximum of 24 hours in the refrigerator. A label with the patient's name and the date is helpful.

Figure 5.6.3
Examples of tube feeds

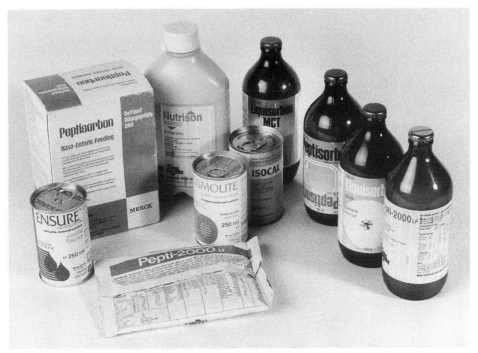

c. Caring for tube-fed patients

In general, it is important to provide information to patients and relatives about the reasons for administering a tube feed. It may also be necessary to convince the patient that this food will supply all the nutrients required.

One bottle of tube feed (Figure 5.6.4) is the equivalent of a complete hot meal. Half a litre contains about 2300 kJ (550 kcal) and 20 grams of protein. This is the equivalent of a meal consisting of five potatoes, 50 grams of meat with gravy or 1 tablespoon of butter, one helping of vegetables, and one carton of full fat yoghurt.

Sometimes it is possible for the patient to drink or eat a little besides the tube feed. When the patient is able and allowed to chew, it is recommended to give something like chewing-gum. This stimulates the production of saliva and can help to prevent inflammation and a bad taste in the mouth.

Study activity 4

a. What kinds of tube feeds are you familiar with?

b. Is it possible for a diabetic patient to be given tube feed?

c. What would you do if you noticed that a tube-fed patient was suffering from diarrhoea?

d. Name three conditions that indicate the use of tube feed.

7. Parenteral feeding

If insufficient nutrients can be absorbed enterally (i.e. through the gastrointestinal tract), nourishment must be given parenterally (via a vein). A major disadvantage of this method is the risk of sepsis. An advantage is that energy-rich feed can be given by passing and therefore 'resting' the gastrointestinal tract.

8. Summary

Food with an altered consistency can provide a solution for people who are unable to chew or swallow normally for physical or psychological reasons, or when normal food is not digested properly. Malnutrition can often be prevented by serving food with an altered consistency.

In this chapter soft foods, liquidised foods, tube feed and parenteral feed were examined. A number of guidelines were given for the care of patients on a diet of food with an altered consistency.

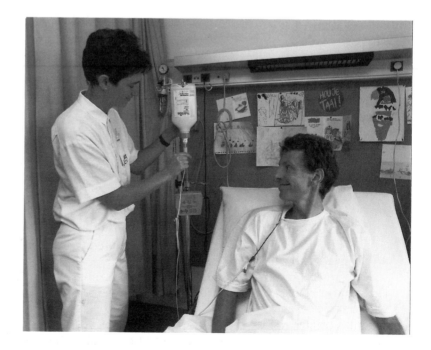

Figure 5.6.4
Bon appétit

Diet and cardiovascular disease

1. Introduction

A large number of people suffer and die from cardiovascular disease, involving arteriosclerosis or stricture of the blood vessels. Such conditions can cause chest pain (angina pectoris) or a myocardial infarction, and in the UK they account for the premature death of around 8% of men and 2% of women. Figure 5.7.1 illustrates rates of myocardial infarction relative to international comparisons.

Chapter 1 of Module 3 examined the importance of diet in the prevention of cardiovascular disease, and this chapter discusses the vital role which diet can play in the treatment of these conditions. It also considers a number of diets which can have a positive effect on risk factors such as hypertension (high blood pressure) and high cholesterol levels in the blood.

Learning outcomes

After studying this chapter the student should be able to:
- describe the sort of lifestyle and dietary behaviour which increases the risk of cardiovascular disease;
- list three factors that increase the risk of hypertension;
- explain briefly what is meant by a low sodium diet;
- suggest two reasons for prescribing a low sodium diet;
- list five foodstuffs which contain a high level of sodium;
- explain what is meant by 'salt substitute' and say when this can be prescribed;
- make four suggestions for an appetising cold meal for a patient on a low sodium diet;
- explain why patients taking diuretics may need special dietary consideration;
- list a number of important points which should be considered when preparing meals for CVA (cerebrovascular accident or stroke) patients;
- provide advice for an appropriate, healthy diet and explain why this kind of diet is recommended for the prevention of cardio-vascular disease;
- describe briefly the kind of diet prescribed for reducing high cholesterol levels in the blood and say when it might be used.

Figure 5.7.1
© The Scotsman 12/7/94

Scots heart-attack rate near top of global league table

by *Bryan Christie*, Health Correspondent

WOMEN in Glasgow have the world's highest rate of heart attacks and are almost nine times more likely to suffer cardiac failure than their counterparts in Spain.

A report published today also shows that Glaswegian women have higher rates than some southern European men, although heart disease has traditionally been seen as a male problem.

A comparison of heart attack rates in 21 countries has confirmed huge international differences, with Scotland at, or close to, the top of the global league table.

Rates among men find those in Glasgow occupying third place behind two provinces in Finland and just in front of Belfast.

The study, reported today in *Circulation*, the journal of the American Heart Association, is based on the largest heart disease research project ever undertaken. The World Health Organisation's Monica project is monitoring patterns of heart disease over a ten-year period in more than 20 million people living across four continents.

Huge international differences have already been found in death rates from heart disease, but the reliability of such statistics has been challenged. Instead, the current study examined the number of people who survived a heart attack between 1985-87 and found that the same differences existed.

Women in Glasgow were well out in front with 256 heart attacks for every 100,000 women, ahead of Belfast (197), Australia (188), Finland (165), France and China (37) and Spain (30). Men in Spain and parts of southern France have lower rates than Scottish women.

High smoking rates among women in Glasgow are thought to lie behind this problem. Other familiar heart disease related problems of high blood pressure and high cholesterol are also common in the city.

Prof Hugh Tunstall-Pedoe, of Dundee University, who led the group which prepared the report, said the lower rates in Mediterranean countries could be due to a diet which relied heavily on fruit and vegetables.

However, he added that the whole question of the precise causes of heart disease remains controversial and the aim of the Monica study is to follow changes in behaviour over time to see if there is a resultant decrease in the amount of heart disease. "We want to find out what the engine is that is driving these changes," he said.

Reductions have already been recorded in rates among men in Finland, but no comparable improvement has been detected in Scotland. Measuring such changes will provide an important indicator to help scientists understand more about heart disease – one of the major killers in the western world.

Prof Tunstall-Pedoe, of the university's cardiovascular epidemiology unit, said the current findings arose out of a remarkable international collaboration which began in the 1980s and united East and West, in spite of difficulties posed by the Cold War.

"The objective of the project is to look next at the reasons why these rates are changing dramatically in different populations. We expect to finalise these results in approximately four years from now but this will depend on the continuation of national and international support during difficult financial times."

The Scottish part of the project has been funded until now by the Scottish Office but indications have been given that future funding may be difficult to obtain. Professor Tunstall-Pedoe said negotiations on this matter are continuing.

2. Risk factors and cardiovascular disease

In most cases, cardiovascular disease is caused by an insufficient flow of blood through the muscle tissue due to stricture of the blood vessels or arteriosclerosis. The process of arteriosclerosis can be influenced by our dietary behaviour and lifestyle, and factors which considerably increase the likelihood of cardiovascular disease are called risk factors. Some of the most important risk factors are:

- high blood pressure (hypertension);
- high cholesterol levels in the blood (hypercholesterolaemia) or other forms of hyperlipidaemia;
- smoking (especially in conjunction with the two factors above);
- insufficient exercise;
- being overweight;
- stress.

Since 1980, the death rate from cardiovascular disease in the UK has decreased slightly, and this may partly be due to improvements in our lifestyle and eating habits. In effect, this means we can take personal responsibility to limit the risks. We can, for instance, exercise regularly, eat a healthy diet and avoid smoking.

Hypertension is very common in the developed countries, where it affects between 8 and 18% of the population. Chronic hypertension can lead to a loss of heart and kidney function, brain haemorrhage or damage to the retina and, while the causes of hypertension are generally unknown, it is clear that high salt consumption, obesity and stress are all contributory factors. Dietary measures can therefore constitute an important part of the treatment (especially since there is, to date, no drug available which will counteract the effects of hypertension on the cardiovascular system).

A high level of cholesterol or of triglycerides in the blood can be caused by eating too much fat, particularly saturated (animal) fat, as well as insufficient mono- or polyunsaturated fat. If arteriosclerosis is not too advanced, a diet with reduced amounts of saturated fats and cholesterol may promote a reduction in the cholesterol level in the blood, and result in a decrease in the risk of cardiovascular disease.

It is worth emphasising that the risk increases greatly when there is a combination of risk factors, for instance when someone with a high cholesterol level also smokes, is under stress, is overweight, or does not take enough exercise.

3. The low sodium diet

Sodium or salt is a mineral that is essential for the body. We find it in blood, sweat, and tears. Salt occurs naturally in nearly all that we eat and drink, even in water. The main source of sodium is table salt (NaCl). In general, there is too much salt in our diet, an average of 2.5 grams a day. Most authorities recommend reducing this intake towards a target, for the year 2000, of 1.6 grams per day (Scotland). Industrially prepared foodstuffs, such as packet foods and canned foods in particular, often have a high salt content.

Reducing the intake of salt may help to lower the blood pressure, but the effectiveness of this varies according to the individual, since one person may be much more sensitive to salt than another. It is likely that other minerals, such as potassium, calcium, and magnesium, also have an adverse effect on blood pressure, so if hypertension has been diagnosed it is important to pay particular attention to diet.

A low sodium diet can be prescribed for two reasons:
- to lower the blood pressure. However, if a patient has high blood pressure and is also overweight, a low energy diet often has more effect on blood pressure than a low salt diet, since attaining a normal body weight is often enough to reduce hypertension;
- to reduce fluid retention, which may occur when there is a decline in heart, liver and kidney function. In such cases, the low sodium diet may be combined with a low fluid intake.

Case study

Mrs Lee is 65 years old. She was widowed a few years ago and has eight grown-up children, all of whom have left home. Since the age of 60, she has suffered heart problems. Two weeks ago she fell, breaking her right leg in two places. She is now in hospital and can only walk with the help of a tripod.

When she was weighed recently it was found that she had gained 2 kg (4.5 lb) over the course of a few days. She weighs 68 kg (10 st 10 lb) and is 168 cm (5 ft 6 in) tall. Mrs Lee complains of being increasingly short of breath. The doctor has diagnosed decompensation cordis.

Because of her gradually worsening heart condition, Mrs Lee will be prescribed a moderately low salt diet to take effect immediately. In general, this means that her hot meals will be cooked without salt and she will not be able to add salt to any of the food she eats.

Study activity 1

a. What do you think caused this patient's weight increase?
b. How would you explain to Mrs Lee why she must maintain a low sodium diet?
c. What would your own reaction be to having to exclude salt from your meals? What suggestions would you make to help someone who only likes salty food?

There are three types of low sodium (Na) diets: no added salt, moderately low sodium, and salt-free.

No Added Salt (NAS) diet is the most frequently prescribed. This means that food should not be salted at the table. Salt is permitted in cooking, but it should be used sparingly. The patient is also advised not to use commercially prepared foodstuffs containing high levels of salt, such as:

– powdered soups, soya sauce, ready-to-serve dishes with meat sauces;
– tinned or packet sauces or soups, powdered gravy mix or gravy cubes;
– sauce mixes for pasta;
– fresh or smoked sausage, hamburgers, smoked ham, or other smoked meats, bacon, pies, and pasties;
– ready-made meals, tinned or frozen;
– crisps, peanuts and other snacks.

Study activity 2

a. Which of the above products do you eat? Discuss the advantages and disadvantages of the products listed.
b. List 10 snacks which are suitable for someone on a NAS diet. What sort of food would be suitable for a visitor to bring to such a patient in hospital?

The restrictions for this modest sodium restriction diet also apply to the moderately low sodium diet (Figure 5.7.2).

A salt-free diet is not often prescribed in practice, but when it is, the use of low salt bread and milk is recommended with this diet. A salt-free diet is occasionally combined with a low fluid diet (around one litre per day), particularly where there is significantly impaired heart function and extensive oedema.

Study activity 3

a. What types of meat used in sandwiches are very salty?
b. Find out which types of cheese contain less salt than ordinary cheddar.

Potassium supplements can reduce hypertension, and potassium levels in the blood can be raised by increasing consumption of fruit and fresh vegetables.

There is a common misconception that sea salt contains less sodium than table salt. Sea salt does, in fact, contain just as much sodium as ordinary table salt, and, therefore, it should not be used as part of a low sodium diet.

a. Special dietary products for a low sodium diet

Just as artificial sweeteners can be used as substitutes for sugar, alternatives to salt are also available. These 'salt substitutes' may contain high levels of potassium and thus present a risk to some patients on a low sodium diet. It is therefore advisable to consult a doctor or dietitian before using these products.

Figure 5.7.2
Examples of the three types of low sodium diet

	No Added Salt diet 80-100 mmol/day (1.8-2.3 g)	Moderate restriction diet 40 mmol/day (1 g)	Salt-free diet 22 mmol/day (0.5 g)
bread	normal	normal	low salt
cheese	normal/lightly salted	low salt*	low salt
ham, etc	normal**	low salt	low salt
sweet fillings	all types	all types	all types
milk and other dairy produce	all types	all types, up to 0.5 l	low salt
hot meals	prepared without salt	prepared without salt	prepared without salt

* Ordinary sandwich fillings can be substituted for fillings lower in salt if salt-free bread is used instead of ordinary bread
** Very salty meat, such as smoked meat, should be avoided

Salt substitutes taste quite different from ordinary salt and do not suit every palate. It is far more sensible to try to adjust to eating food without salt because salt-free meals can be made just as tasty as salted food by the addition of herbs and spices and by varying the methods of preparation.

Salt-reduced dietary products (Figure 5.7.3) carry labels such as 'low sodium', 'for a low sodium diet', 'unsalted', 'no salt added' or 'low salt'. Mineral salt is also sold as a substitute for table salt but, although much of the sodium in it has been replaced by other minerals, it still contains too much sodium to qualify as an item for a low sodium diet.

b. Practical hints for a low sodium diet
We normally use salt out of habit, having acquired the taste for it from a very young age. Adding a lot of salt to our food diminishes our sense of taste as salt impairs the functioning of the mucous membrane and the taste buds. A low sodium diet, therefore, can allow a patient to recover a well-developed sense of taste.
Some tips for low sodium cold meals
–   Low salt bread dries out very quickly, so it is important to store it properly and not to prepare sandwiches too far in advance;

–   The flavour of low salt sandwiches can be improved by using lettuce, cucumber, radishes, tomatoes, fresh fruit, herbs or low salt mustard;
–   Home-made salt-free meat loaf can be delicious in sandwiches;
–   Low salt brown or wholemeal bread has more flavour than white;
–   Low salt milk can be flavoured by adding instant coffee, cocoa, or fruit syrup.
Some tips for low sodium hot meals
–   Fresh herbs, spices and lemon juice can add zest to a meal.
–   Cook or steam vegetables quickly in very little water so they retain their flavour.

c. Other aspects of the low sodium diet
Long-term hypertension is a potentially dangerous condition, and prompt treatment is very important. Patients often underestimate its severity because its direct consequences are not immediately noticeable. The low sodium diet makes an immediate and significant impact on their lives, and therefore there is a danger that it will not be strictly adhered to. Consequently, it is vital that health care workers provide sound information and constant support to hypertensive patients. It is usually easier to encourage patients to

Figure 5.7.3
Products with varying amounts of salt

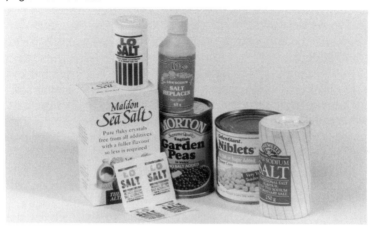

maintain a low salt diet once they have realised, either through explanation, or personal experience, how the body responds to digestion of salt by retaining fluid.

When patients have been prescribed diuretics, it is recommended that they take extra fruit, fruit juice, potatoes, or fresh vegetables. This is because diuretics encourage the loss of high levels of potassium through the urine, and a potassium deficiency can cause impaired cardiac function.

One of the possible consequences of hypertension is a brain haemorrhage (cerebrovascular accident or CVA). Most patients who have suffered a CVA do not need a special diet, but additional factors or complications such as being overweight, hypertension, diabetes mellitus, difficulties with swallowing and constipation may necessitate dietary advice.

Patients who are comatose following a CVA will be fed by tube, with a change to a liquid diet when consciousness is regained. Temporary problems with swallowing are often encountered at this point, and thick liquids such as yoghurt and thin porridge will be easier to drink than thin ones such as tea, coffee, water and fruit juices, although thickening these drinks with cornflour or commercial thickening agents may provide a solution.

For hemiplegic patients, eating with-

out assistance is often very difficult, and specially adapted tableware may prove useful. A CVA patient's total intake of fluids should be closely monitored, since there may be a tendency to avoid drinking if going to the toilet is presenting problems.

4. Diet, hypercholesterolaemia, and hyperlipidaemia

In view of the widespread incidence of cardiovascular disease, Britain's entire population can be considered a high risk group. Advice about maintaining a healthy diet, taking sufficient exercise, and not smoking is therefore vital for everyone. As far as diet is concerned, the advice given in Chapter 2 of Module 2 is recommended for anyone in Britain over five years old, but it will be especially important for:

– people with a serum cholesterol level between 5 and 6.5 mmol/l;
– people who have a higher than average level of triglycerides in the blood.

If the serum cholesterol level is 6.5 mmol/l or higher, or when there is another form of hyperlipidaemia, a stricter diet with greater restrictions on saturated fats will be necessary (see Figures 5.7.4 and 5.7.5 and the advice and suggestions given below). Practically, this means recommending low fat and semi-skimmed dairy products, low fat cheese and lean meat. An increased intake of unsaturated fatty acids

Figure 5.7.4
Some of the foodstuffs in an average diet and recommended alternatives for reducing the serum cholesterol level

Average diet	*Recommended alternatives to reduce serum cholesterol*
full cream dairy products	low fat and semi-skimmed dairy products
full fat cheese	low fat cheese
meat products with an average fat content	lean meat products
margarine/butter	low fat diet margarine (at least 60% polyunsaturated fat)
vegetables, fruit, pulses	more vegetables, fruit, pulses
bread	more bread and other wholemeal products
sugar	less sugar

is also recommended, and this can be achieved using low fat or diet margarine (with a minimum of 60% polyunsaturated fats), oils such as sunflower oil, corn oil, soya bean or olive oil, a moderate intake of peanuts and other nuts, and fatty fish.

Finally, it should be noted that being overweight constitutes an additional risk factor for the development and progression of arteriosclerosis. Most authorities consider a body weight with a QI of between 20 and 25 to be ideal (see Chapter 4 of Module 3). Losing weight usually has a beneficial effect on the serum cholesterol level and on the blood pressure.

Dietary advice and suggestions for reducing the cholesterol level
Cold meal
- brown or wholemeal bread thinly spread with low fat margarine with lean meat, low fat cheese, or peanut butter or fresh fruit
- no more than 3-4 eggs per week
- vegetable salad
- low fat or semi-skimmed milk products

Hot meal
- potatoes (or an appropriate alternative)
- vegetables
- lean meat or fish (or an appropriate

alternative)
- liver or kidney not more than once a fortnight
- fry and bake with sunflower oil or diet margarine, which can also be used for gravy or sauce
- desserts made with low fat or semi-skimmed dairy products

Snacks
- coffee/tea
- scone or digestive biscuit with low fat margarine
- fresh fruit or a handful of nuts
- low fat or semi-skimmed dairy products

Study activity 4

a. The advice and suggestions above encourage increased consumption of vegetables and decreased consumption of meat products. Why do you think this is?
b. Why is low fat cheese recommended?
c. Name five types of lean meat or meat products which could be used in sandwiches suitable for someone with a high cholesterol level.

Figure 5.7.5
Serum cholesterol levels

Serum cholesterol level	Dietary advice
lower than 5 mmol/l (normal)	maintain a nutritional, well-balanced diet
5.0-6.4 mmol/l (slightly high)	maintain a nutritional, well-balanced diet
6.5-7.9 mmol/l (high)	adopt a special diet to reduce cholesterol level, with medication if necessary
8 mmol/l or over (very high)	adopt a special diet to reduce cholesterol level, with medication if necessary, then have a further assessment after 3 months

Case Study

A 43-year-old man was admitted to the cardiology ward after suffering a major heart attack. His serum cholesterol level was recorded as 8 mmol/l. The dietitian was consulted and, whilst taking a dietary history, she was astounded when the patient told her that he ate at least two eggs a day. This, he said, was partly because he liked eggs, and partly because he had six hens who were all good layers, and it would be a shame to waste the eggs!

The British Heart Foundation (see Appendix 3) provides advice and information on heart disease to the general public and supports research in the field of cardiovascular disease. The foundation publishes a series of free booklets on various aspects of cardivascular conditions and these are available from hospitals, surgeries and health centres throughout the United Kingdom.

5. Summary

Certain lifestyles and dietary behaviour can increase the risk of cardiovascular disease and diet can also play a vital role in the treatment of such disorders. For example, a reduced salt intake is often prescribed for hypertension or fluid retention. However, when a hypertensive patient is also overweight, a low energy intake will be a major criterion of the diet.

Three types of low sodium diet were discussed: the salt-free diet, the moderately low sodium diet and the No Added Salt diet. The latter is the most frequently prescribed. A number of guidelines and hints for preparing appetising salt-free meals were given.

A high level of cholesterol in the blood is one of the risk factors for cardiovascular disease. It is sometimes possible to lower the cholesterol level by maintaining an appropriate diet. If the body weight is also excessive, losing weight can have a beneficial impact as it can cause the cholesterol level to fall.

Diet and kidney disease

1. Introduction

Although the quantity and the composition of our meals vary from day to day, the amount of water and salts in our body remains essentially constant. It is mainly the kidneys which maintain this salt/water balance by removing superfluous substances such as minerals, water and the toxic degradation products derived from the breaking down of proteins. If renal function is impaired, nausea, loss of appetite and itchiness can result. Oedema or hypertension can also develop when the kidneys do not excrete enough water or salts. These symptoms and conditions can be largely managed by dietary measures, but a diet designed to cope with impaired renal function is often quite drastic. It is therefore especially important for patients to be fully informed about the reasons for their diet, and about the opportunities for variation and choice.

All the blood in a healthy body passes through the kidneys once every 5-7 minutes in a system of continual filtration which removes superfluous and toxic substances. These are then excreted in the urine. The composition of our blood is determined not only by what we eat but also, to a large extent, by what the kidneys excrete.

The position of the kidneys is shown in Figure 5.8.1.

Learning outcomes

After studying this chapter the student should be able to:
- explain why a low protein diet may be prescribed in the case of impaired renal function;
- explain which factors determine the degree of protein restriction in the diet;
- explain why a low protein diet should contain more carbohydrates and fats than an average diet;
- list five foodstuffs which cannot be used without restriction in a low protein diet, and five foodstuffs which can;
- state when and why special low protein dietary products must be used in a low protein diet;
- explain why a low potassium diet may be prescribed in the case of impaired renal function;
- outline the circumstances in which a low fluid diet is necessary;

– explain what determines the quantity of fluids permitted in a diet;
– state two important considerations in planning the diet of a patient with impaired renal function;
– understand the most important dietary measures for preventing the formation of kidney stones.

2. Dietary modification in kidney failure

The most common diets prescribed for kidney disease are:
– the low protein diet
– the low sodium diet
– the low potassium diet
– the fluid restricted diet
– the low phosphate diet

Figure 5.8.1
1 The kidneys

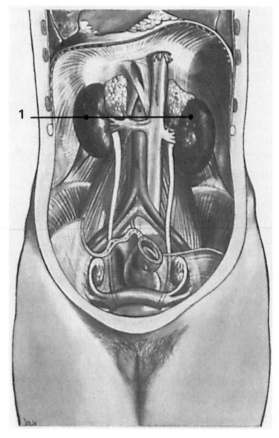

Patients with deterioration of kidney function often require a combination of these diets. In general, the diet includes a daily menu in which the permitted quantities of protein, sodium, potassium, and fluid have been calculated. The dietitian gradually teaches the patient to keep within these dietary guidelines, and monitors the effects of the diet on the patient's biochemistry (for example, by measuring the levels of urea, creatinine, sodium, phosphate, calcium and potassium in a sample of the patient's blood and urine) so that adjustments to the dietary guidelines may be made if necessary.

a. Early intervention with a modified diet
Dietary protein restriction has long been recognised as an effective treatment in renal failure. However, evidence is accumulating that preservation of renal function may be achieved by *early* restriction of dietary protein, that is, before the patient becomes symptomatic (Figure 5.8.2).

b. The low protein diet
Degradation products such as urea are derived from protein digestion and eliminated in the urine. When the kidney function becomes impaired, insufficient excretion of these products occurs and this leads to a build-up in the level of urea in the blood (uraemia). The resulting symptoms include nausea, vomiting, itchiness and loss of appetite. As soon as the dietary intake of protein is reduced, however, urea levels in the blood fall and the symptoms start to disappear.

In certain cases, such as men suffering from glomerulonephritis, the deterioration of the kidneys can be decelerated by prescribing a low protein diet at an early stage. There are several factors which determine

Figure 5.8.2
© Sunday Express 1993

Diet change that may save kidneys

Neville Hodgkinson

PREVENTIVE MEDICINE is often misinterpreted as meaning a need to take pills to stave off illness. But the best kinds of prevention are those that free patients from the need for any kind of treatment.

One group who often do not receive appropriate help in this respect are those with damaged kidneys. Many enter a downward spiral, leading eventually to a life on a kidney machine, without being told about lifestyle changes that could halt their decline.

The kidneys have about a million functional units each, known as nephrons, with which to do their job of excreting waste products and maintaining a proper balance in body fluids.

As soon as a certain proportion of these have been destroyed, the rest are more easily overburdened. If nothing is done, the disease becomes progressive. There are more than 2,500 new chronic cases of this kind every year in the UK.

But it makes good sense to believe that by reducing the toxic load the kidneys have to handle, such as by cutting down on rich food, the decline can be slowed or even halted. Suggestions to this effect were first made more than 40 years ago.

But many specialists have been loath to acknowledge the role of diet in the disease.

An exception has been a group at Guy's Hospital, London, where for some years doctors have been advising diabetic patients with failing kidneys either to eat less protein generally, or to switch from meat to vegetable protein, or both.

Now Australian doctors have reported scientific evidence of dramatic benefits in kidney patients put on a low protein diet.

Only two out of 31 patients who were switched on to such a diet at the Royal Melbourne Hospital went on to develop kidney failure – necessitating dialysis treatment or a transplant – compared with nine out of a comparable group of 33 patients who carried on eating their usual diet.

In the "normal diet" group, almost all showed a substantial reduction in kidney efficiency over the 18 months of the study, whereas on average the low protein group declined hardly at all. Anyone with a kidney problem should take these findings to heart.

---

the degree of protein restriction necessary in the diet, including:

- the severity of the uraemia;
- the degree of renal impairment (this can be assessed by measuring the creatinine level in the blood);
- the type of dialysis used, if any.

The greater the disturbance in kidney function, the more restricted the intake of protein must be. It is impossible, however, to exclude protein entirely from the diet, as protein substances in the body are essential to its structure and function.

The intake of foods containing high levels of protein, such as meat, fish, cheese, eggs, nuts, dairy produce, and pulses needs to be restricted, even in modest protein-restricted diets (0.75 g of protein per kilogram of body weight per day). When the impairment of kidney function demands a moderately low or a very low protein diet (0.5 g or 0.3 g of protein per kilogram of body weight per day), even foods with a lower protein content, such as bread, potatoes, rice, and biscuits, can only be consumed in small quantities.

A low protein diet is different for every individual. The extent to which a patient's kidneys still function, or the patient's dialysis, must naturally be considered, as must his or her personal tastes and preferences. As a result of the protein restriction, the diet needs to have a higher fat and carbohydrate content in order to provide sufficient energy. If a shortage of energy occurs, the body starts to break down its own protein to make up the shortfall. This causes the formation of urea which is exactly what the diet is designed to prevent. Foods which will provide energy in the form of fats and carbohydrates include butter, margarine, oils, cream, sugar, jam, honey, fruit, fruit juice and vegetables.

Case study

Mr Dean is 66 years old. He is 170 cm (5 ft 7 in) tall and weighs 84 kg (13 st 3 lb). He is a bachelor and lives with his sister and her husband. Until he retired last year, he was a lorry driver, and in his final year at work he often felt very tired, but he attributed this to hard work. Over the past few months he has been suffering from frequent nausea and vomiting, and his appetite is depressed. He has lost almost 6.5 kg (14 lb) over the last two months. He was examined by a specialist who diagnosed uraemia, caused by inflammation of the kidneys, and recommended a low protein diet. Consequently, the dietitian in consultation with Mr Dean has now compiled the following diet:

Breakfast
- 1 slice of brown toast with butter
- 1 portion of marmalade
- 1 small bowl of cereal with milk
- 1 boiled egg
- tea with sugar

Morning snack
- coffee with sugar (and some cream)
- 1 scone with butter
- 1 piece of fruit

Lunch
- 50g of meat (or equivalent)
- 1 spoonful of gravy
- 1 serving of vegetables
- 3 potatoes
- 1 bowl of vanilla ice cream

Afternoon snack
- tea with sugar
- 1 glass of apple juice
- 1 cracker generously spread with butter and jam, or honey

Dinner
- small bowl of plain boiled pasta
- small serving of bolognaise sauce
- small green salad
- tea with sugar
- glass of milk

Supper
- coffee with sugar (and some cream)
- 1 cracker spread thickly with butter, jam, or honey
- 1 glass of fruit juice

Study activity 1

a. Calculate the amount of protein in this daily menu.
b. How much protein per day would Mr Dean normally need?
c. Why are small meals that are rich in energy especially appropriate in this situation?
d. Is Mr Dean allowed to freely omit the foods containing protein from his menu?
e. Think of some snacks that do not contain protein that can therefore be eaten freely.
f. Why is butter spread generously in this diet?
g. What can Mr Dean do if he does not want his milk at dinner?

Special dietary products for a low protein diet

In a low protein diet it is possible to substitute special low protein products for foods such as bread, pasta, and cake. Such products include: low protein bread, bread mix, crackers, spaghetti, macaroni, French toast, and biscuits (Figure 5.8.3). They contain negligible levels of protein or else none at all, so they can be consumed without restriction. There are some disadvantages of these products including the flavour (the products are sometimes fairly unpalatable) and the high price, but they are, nevertheless, indispensable for people who require a high intake of energy but who must maintain a low protein diet.

Although sugar may not be a recommended component of a healthy diet, it is often included in a low protein diet in order to provide sufficient energy.

Study activity 2

Mr Dean feels hungry and would like some more bread. What would you recommend?

c. The low sodium diet

When the body is unable to excrete enough water and salt because of impaired kidney function, oedema and hypertension may result. In this situation, a low sodium diet is often prescribed, with the degree of restriction of the sodium intake depending on the severity of the disease. The three types of low sodium diet were discussed in the previous chapter.

d. The low potassium diet

Loss of kidney function can also lead to insufficient secretion of potassium, causing hyperkalaemia, which can lead to irregular heartbeat and cardiac arrest (acute heart death). To prevent this, patients with severe renal impairment or who undergo haemodialysis treatment will require a low potassium diet. This means that the intake of foods rich in potassium, such as fruit, fruit juices, potatoes, other vegetables, and dairy products must be restricted. Potassium restriction is usually implemented when serum potassium levels exceed 5.0 mmol/l. The use of salt substitutes which contain a high proportion of potassium is therefore strongly discouraged.

e. The low fluid diet

When a patient with a kidney disorder produces little or no urine, restriction of the fluid intake will be necessary. The amount of fluid that can be given depends on the degree of renal impairment, and keeping an accurate record of the fluid balance in the body is imperative in such cases. All fluid intake, which includes all drinks, soup, fruit and desserts, must be recorded and it is important not to overlook any liquid taken with medication. A restricted fluid intake is usually very difficult for the patient, but there are numerous ways of facilitating the situation. These include:

– using small cups and glasses for drinks;
– freezing drinks into ice cubes;
– giving sour drinks (which quench the thirst) rather than sweet drinks (which stimulate thirst).

For patients on haemodialysis, fluid intake should be calculated according to urine output as well as the frequency of dialysis.

Figure 5.8.3
Low protein dietary products

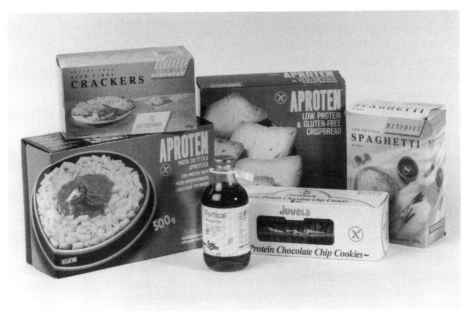

f. The low phosphate diet

In the kidneys, there is a network of capillaries called the glomeruli. These act as filtering units for the blood. Water and salts that are surplus to the body's requirements, together with waste products from the body, are filtered by the glomeruli from the fluid passing through the kidneys to be excreted as urine, whilst a solution of salts that are useful to the body is returned to the blood from the fluid. The glomeruli have an important function in our bodies, not only in the purification of our blood but also in the regulation of the balance of salts in the blood.

In advanced kidney disease, however, the glomeruli can become affected so that their function of purification and salt regulation becomes impaired. Consequently, phosphate is retained and the calcium/phosphate ratio may become disturbed. Since calcium and phosphorus combine in the body to form calcium phosphate (the hard material in our bones and teeth), an appropriate ratio of calcium and phosphorus must be maintained. If not, bone disease could result as sometimes happens in advanced kidney disease.

This disturbance in salt regulation caused by the glomeruli's inability to perform their regulatory function may result in an excess of phosphate in the blood. In such a case (usually when the plasma phosphate concentration exceeds 2.0 mmol/l), dietary intake of phosphorus may have to be restricted, and a low phosphate diet prescribed. Such a diet usually means restricting the intake of phosphorus to below 700 mg/day.

Intake of foods such as wholemeal products and dairy produce is restricted. Care must be taken not to compromise the intake of calcium since this would further disturb the calcium/phosphate ratio. Patients are therefore encouraged to reach a calcium intake of 1,000 mg/day. The use of phosphate-binding agents, such as calcium carbonate or aluminium hydroxide, may also reduce phosphate levels. Calcium carbonate is now preferred as it causes fewer toxicity problems.

3. Renal replacement therapy

When a patient reaches end-stage kidney failure, medical intervention with renal replacement therapy is required to preserve life. The options for treatment are dialysis or transplantation.

Two principal modes of dialysis currently available are haemodialysis and peritoneal dialysis:

Haemodialysis (HD) requires the use of an artificial kidney or dialyser where the patient has two or three weekly sessions of intermittent dialysis either at home or in a renal unit.

Peritoneal dialysis is effected through the patient's peritoneum, the dialysing solution being introduced into and removed from the peritoneal cavity. It can be either intermittent, with sessions of dialysis over the week, or continuous (Continuous Ambulatory Peritoneal Dialysis, or CAPD).

Peritoneal dialysis is the preferred method because dialysis is continuous and this prevents some symptoms that occur between dialysis sessions in the cases of haemodialysis and intermittent peritoneal dialysis. These symptoms include electrolyte imbalance, fluid overload, and alteration in the levels of the various blood components. The reduction in symptoms thus improves the quality of life of the patient undergoing this type of dialysis.

Since both modes of dialysis have been shown to be catabolic (i.e. aggravate muscle breakdown), high protein intakes are required (for HD, 1-1.2 g/kg of ideal body weight per day and for CAPD, 1.2-1.5 g/kg of ideal body weight per day). Prescription of other nutrients depends on the mode of dialysis, the patient's biochemistry, and medication.

The transplant patient's diet is essentially normal; however, the use of steroids may aggravate the development of obesity.

4. Caring for patients with impaired renal function

One of the chief problems in the care of kidney patients is that they are often seriously ill, with no appetite and frequent feelings of nausea. Such patients will experience difficulty in maintaining a low protein (or possibly an even more restricted) diet.

It is very important for patients and their families to be adequately informed about the reasons for the diet and the variations which are possible within it. Food can be served in smaller portions and more frequently, and extra attention to the appearance and temperature of the food may help to encourage the patient to eat it.

In cases of severe renal impairment, supplements of calcium, iron, vitamins of the B complex, and vitamin C may be necessary. If any potassium-based medication is administered, it must be taken in combination with foods containing protein.

The Kidney Patients' Association provides support for patients treated by dialysis or who have undergone transplantation, as well as those being managed by diet or undergoing therapy for kidney stones. The Kidney Foundation, a registered charity, also supports research into kidney disease (see Appendix 3).

5. Kidney stones

Kidney stones are relatively common. They occur about twice as frequently in men as in women and, in most cases, the cause of stone formation is unknown. It has been established that diet does play a role and, in particular, that the risk of stone formation is reduced by frequent drinks totalling 2-3 litres of fluid per day.

Kidney stones can be composed of various substances, although in about 90% of cases they contain calcium. Where calcium stones are present, moderation in the intake of foods containing calcium is advised. These include milk, cheese, yoghurt and milk-based desserts. In addition, an increased intake of high fibre diet is recommended as this may help to reduce the absorption of calcium.

A diet which contains reduced levels of calcium but normal levels of oxalate (a substance found chiefly in vegetables and ordinary tea) may actually increase the likelihood of kidney stone formation. The oxalate level must also be reduced and this means limiting the intake of foods rich in oxalate, such as spinach, rhubarb, mushrooms, chocolate, cola and strong tea. Vitamin C supplements should also be stopped. Herbal teas are low in oxalate and so make a good alternative to ordinary tea.

6. Summary

People suffering from kidney disorders may experience nausea, loss of appetite and itchiness. Symptoms such as fluid retention and hypertension may also be apparent. Certain dietary measures can significantly reduce these symptoms.

This chapter discussed the low protein, low sodium, low potassium, low fluid, and low phosphate diets. The more kidney function is impaired, the greater the need for dietary restriction. Consequently, with a low protein diet, sufficient energy intake is important. A low protein diet should contain more carbohydrates and products high in fats than a normal diet. Special low protein dietary products are used when necessary.

For patients who have undergone renal replacement therapy, some dietary adjustment may be necessary depending on the type of therapy used. Patients with kidney disorders are often seriously ill and suffer from nausea and loss of appetite.

The chapter ended by discussing the relationship between diet and the formation of some types of kidney stones.

Diet and cancer

1. Introduction

In Western society cancer is, after heart and arterial disease, the second most prevalent cause of death, and the incidence is increasing. This is partly due to the aging of the population since cancer primarily affects older people, but the incidence is increasing for all age groups. In Chapter 1 of Module 3, the possible connections between diet and the development of cancer were examined. Here we will examine the role which diet may play once cancer has been diagnosed. In general, a specially adapted diet can improve a patient's fitness and quality of life, and enable him or her to cope better with the various therapies which are available. Some alternative practitioners believe that cancer can even be cured with the appropriate diet, and the Bristol diet is probably the most well-known example of this.

Learning outcomes

After studying this chapter the student should be able to:
- list three causes of dietary problems in cancer patients;
- explain why appropriate nutrition can benefit a cancer patient;
- list some dietary measures which will alleviate common problems such as a dry mouth, a painful mouth or throat, nausea, vomiting and depressed appetite;
- offer a personal opinion of the Bristol Diet, taking into account both its nutritional value and its practicality;
- understand in which areas particular attention is needed in the care of cancer patients.

2. Dietary problems and cancer

Cancer patients frequently have poor nutritional status, and there is often noticeable weight loss. In many cases they eat very little because chewing, swallowing, or digesting food is hindered by a tumour in the mouth, throat, oesophagus, or stomach. Surgery and radiotherapy can also cause problems, as can treatment with cytotoxic drugs used in chemotherapy which slow down the rate of cell division. Such procedures may cause pain, reduce the production of saliva, and alter or depress the sense of taste. It sometimes happens that a patient suddenly dislikes a food which has always been a favourite. Chemotherapy or radiotherapy treatment is often accompanied by symptoms like nausea and vomiting. In addition, psychological factors such as uncertainty and fear can diminish the appetite.

Case study

Mrs Spencer is 47 years old. Six months ago she underwent a hysterectomy as the result of the discovery of a carcinoma, and she is now undergoing chemotherapy on an outpatient basis. She spends one day every three weeks undergoing treatment, and on these days she feels so sick that she can hardly eat at all. She only ever manages a little yoghurt with fruit. She still feels nauseated when going home at night, and the feeling diminishes only gradually over the days following treatment. She tries to eat as healthily as possible between treatments in order to be fit in time for her next session, but she suffers periods of depression which make this difficult.

A good nutritional status is an important consideration in cancer patients. In practice, a patient's nutritional status is often ignored until the disease is too far advanced for diet to be of much help, but malnutrition can greatly aggravate the patient's condition. A well-nourished patient, however, will feel more fit, both physically and mentally, and suffer less from complications and side-effects of treatment. If a patient loses too much weight or is undernourished, it might even be necessary to cease radiotherapy or chemotherapy treatment. In addition, an appropriate diet will help the patient to recover more rapidly after treatment.

3. Dietary recommendations for cancer patients

a. Common dietary recommendations
Normally, the dietary recommendations for cancer patients are simply aimed at maintaining or attaining good nutritional status. A healthy diet based on the food guide could be used as the starting point.

However, the diet should always be adapted to the patient's individual symptoms and preferences as much as possible (Figure 5.9.1).

In practice, it is often very difficult for the patient to eat enough. The times at which a person is hungry do not always coincide with meal times in a hospital or nursing home, and special attention is therefore required from the nursing staff in this respect. Where appetite is poor or there is undernourishment, a diet high in energy and protein is recommended. (Practical guidelines for such a diet are given in Chapter 3 of this module.) Depending on the circumstances and the patient's preferences, a liquidised diet or tube feed may be appropriate.

Study activity 1

What would you recommend for a patient who no longer wants hot meals? He has said that even the smell of the food makes him nauseated, and he has far fewer problems with cold meals.

b. The Bristol Diet
The established methods of treating cancer include surgery, radiotherapy and chemotherapy, and often two or all three methods are combined. These methods are based on the belief that cancer is a 'localised disease', and they assume that once the tumour is removed the patient will recover. Over the years, these forms of treatment have continued to improve in efficiency and now almost half of the people who develop cancer can be cured by them.

A number of cancer patients turn to complementary medicine (Figure 5.9.2), and one of the most well-known complementary therapies is the Bristol Diet (Figure 5.9.3), first introduced in the 1980s. Dr Alec Forbes, a consultant physician in Plymouth, believed that cancer could not occur in a healthy body that had a healthy metabolism. He saw it, not as a localised disease of cell mutations, but rather as a disease of the entire body which occurs due to deficiencies in a number of essential nutrients. The Bristol Diet combines an individually adapted diet with a number of supplementary substances, particularly vitamins and minerals. The foods used in the diet are produced without chemical aids and have undergone the minimum processing possible. The diet diverges considerably from our normal eating patterns, and many people find it difficult to adapt to life without coffee, meat, sugar and tobacco.

Figure 5.9.1
Possible dietary solutions to some of the common problems experienced by cancer patients

Problem	Dietary recommendations
Dry mouth	Keep the mouth moist by frequently taking small sips of liquid Take drinks with meals, and a lot of gravy or sauce Eat porridge instead of bread Chew sugar-free gum Suck peppermints or lemon drops For sandwich fillings, use foods such as well-cooked meat or scrambled egg
Painful mouth or throat due to inflammation of the mucous membrane	Exclude sharp spices or herbs from the diet Exclude sour, very salty or sweet products Avoid drinks which are either too hot or too cold Avoid citrus fruits, which can irritate the mucous membranes; eat fruits such as bananas, peaches, pears and strawberries since they are less acidic Sour products such as yoghurt, fruit salad and fruit juices can be given a milder taste by adding some cream
Difficulty in swallowing due to presence of mucus	Take sips of water Camomile tea, brown ale or stout, pineapple juice, and fizzy mineral water will dissolve mucus The production of watery saliva can be stimulated by chewing and by sour substances (see Chapter 6 of this module)
Nausea and vomiting vomiting	Drink plenty, since lack of fluids aggravates the feeling of nausea Sufficient liquid intake can also compensate for fluid lost through Take smaller, more frequent meals Get as much fresh air as possible Sometimes cold dishes appeal more than hot ones
Poor appetite	See the recommendations in Chapter 3 of this module

*If necessary, consult a dietitian for recommendations which could be adapted to the individual patient for each of these problems.

Figure 5.9.2
© The Scotsman 8/7/94

Cancer sufferers seek alternative remedies

by *Bryan Christie*, Health Correspondent

CANCER patients are turning increasingly to unorthodox treatments to help them cope with the disease.

A study of patients at two Lothian hospitals has found that one patient in six used complementary therapies such as mental imagery, spiritual or faith healing, special diets and vitamin supplements.

Although such treatments did not have any proven effects in combating the cancer, they helped to improve the outlook of patients, making them more optimistic about their condition.

A report on the study, published today in the *British Medical Journal*, says that women from middle-class backgrounds are most likely to use complementary therapies.

Dr Maurice Slevin, a consultant oncologist at St Bartholomew's Hospital, who worked on the study, said "One of the main findings of this study was the importance of giving cancer patients a sense of hope.

"If they do not get it from their doctor, they may seek it from complementary practitioners. Doctors and nurses need to establish good communication and maintain an optimistic attitude with patients."

If the patient has no appetite, the Bristol Diet recommends that, for a few weeks only fruit, fruit juices, vegetables, or vegetable juices be taken. This promotes the detoxification of the body and improves the physical and spiritual condition of the patient, so that the appetite will return naturally. Despite the fact that current medical science takes a negative view of the Bristol Diet, it appeals to some cancer patients, especially those for whom mainstream medical practice can offer little hope.

The Bristol Diet may sometimes be a last resort, but it is often also the choice of patients who want to make an active contribution to their own healing process rather than simply be the passive subject of therapy. It does, however, require great motivation on the part of the patient because of the often drastic changes in eating habits which the diet demands.

To date, the Bristol Diet has not been studied enough to allow a fair evaluation of its worth. Some patients become well again after following it, but there are also many examples of remarkable cures with other more common treatments. Nevertheless, doctors who apply the Bristol Diet are of the unanimous opinion that the well-being of the patient does improve, that there is less pain, and that patients look better.

Study activity 2

A 65-year-old man has had leukaemia for a year and he is undergoing chemotherapy. During his treatment sessions and for a short time afterwards, he suffers from nausea, vomiting and sometimes diarrhoea. In the periods between treatments, he feels much better. Recently, some friends told him about the Bristol Diet after reading about some of its convincing results.

a. This patient tells you that he would like to try the Bristol Diet. How would you react?

b. What is your own opinion of the Bristol Diet? Evaluate its nutritional value, its practicality (at home or in a hospital or nursing home), and its cost. How might it infringe upon medical ethics?

c. Explain in your own words why good nutritional status is important for this patient.

Figure 5.9.3
The Bristol Diet

Take daily: – 0.5-1 litre of buttermilk
            – wholemeal bread
            – butter, hard cheese
            – 2 raw egg yolks
            – fresh vegetables (possibly in the form of juice)
            – fresh fruit, particularly citrus fruit (possibly in the form of juice)
            – unpolished rice
            – pulses

Do not take: – sugar or flour
            – meat or fish, or stock made from meat or fish
            – egg white
            – margarine
            – baked foods
            – coffee, tea, cocoa, yoghurt, water, soft drinks or alcohol
            – vegetables of the cabbage family
            – mushrooms, asparagus or rhubarb
            – potatoes
            – legumes

c. Working with cancer patients
As well as ensuring that a cancer patient has a diet adapted to his individual needs, the health care worker also has to consider the psychological and social consequences of the disease. Patients often do not want to eat because of their feelings of fear and insecurity. Nursing staff can help enormously by showing a positive attitude and by taking the time to discuss the illness with the patients.

Families are also likely to be distressed and bringing food is often the only way they can think of to express their concern. However, forcing food on people is always pointless, and it may actually achieve the opposite of the desired effect. By discussing the problems as fully as possible with the relevant people, solutions can usually be found which help to alleviate suffering and which take account of the patient's wishes and requirements.

4. Summary

Short-term and long-term dietary problems are both common amongst cancer patients. Appetite can be impaired by various factors, including the treatment itself, feelings of insecurity, and fear, which make weight loss common. Unfortunately, in practice, a patient's nutritional status may well be ignored until the disease is too advanced for dietary change to have much effect.

There are many advantages of ensuring the patient is adequately nourished. He will feel fitter, both physically and mentally, and will suffer less from the side-effects and complications of treatment. Dietary solutions have been suggested for some of the common problems which affect cancer patients, and the Bristol Diet has also been discussed.

Food allergies and food intolerance 10

1. Introduction

The spread of pollen from grass, cereals, flowers, or trees causes a blocked nose, fits of sneezing, watering and itchy eyes, earache, fatigue and shortness of breath in many people. These are all symptoms of 'hay fever', which is caused by an allergy to the pollen of certain plants. There are thousands of other substances which can cause allergic reactions, and many of them are present in foods.

Food is associated with two distinct types of allergic reactions: food allergy and food intolerance. In cases of food allergy, the body's immune system produces antibodies against some particular substances which are present in the food, and the result is an allergic reaction. In food intolerance, the immune system is not activated but the food itself causes the allergic reaction.

In both cases, the therapy appears to be simple: find the food which causes the symptoms and stop eating it. However, tracing the substance that causes the reaction can sometimes be quite difficult.

Learning outcomes

After studying this chapter the student should be able to:
- list four symptoms which could indicate a food allergy or food intolerance;
- list five foods or food components which often cause food allergy or food intolerance;
- name two techniques for tracing the cause of food allergy or food intolerance;
- describe the therapy which is generally applied in cases of allergic reaction to food.

2. The symptoms of food hypersensitivity

The symptoms associated with allergic reactions vary greatly, and every patient has his own distinctive pattern. These symptoms can be localised in the skin, the gastrointestinal tract or the respiratory passages, and they may even be of a neurological nature. The skin, for example, may show signs of eczema and hives. In the gastrointestinal tract, the intestinal mucous membrane can be affected resulting in stomach pains and diarrhoea. Other gastrointestinal reactions may include nausea and vomiting. The respiratory passages can display a range of symptoms reminiscent of a chronic cold, bronchitis, other chest infections, or asthma. Neurological symptoms include changes in behaviour (such as hyperactivity and depression), migraine headaches and problems with co-ordination. Some people consider rheumatism to be an allergic reaction too.

Some of the symptoms which can be caused by allergic reactions are:

Gastrointestinal tract
nausea and vomiting
reduced appetite
stomachache
diarrhoea or constipation or both
Respiratory passages
inflammation of the middle ear
rhinitis
chronic coughing
bronchitis
asthma
Skin
nappy dermatitis
atopic dermatitis
urticaria
angio-oedema
oedema of the lips
Blood and circulation
anaemia
hypoproteinaemia
anaphylactic shock
Central nervous system
hypertonia
excessive weeping
irritability
headache and migraine
General
fatigue
fear
concentration problems
aches in the muscles and joints
headaches

Case study

Susan, 21 years old: 'Even when I was a baby, I showed symptoms of hypersensitivity. I often suffered from stomach cramps and eczema, and I cried a lot. However, 20 years ago these symptoms were not recognised by GPs. As a child I often suffered from migraines and was given medication for this but it didn't help. Gradually the symptoms became worse. When I was 18 years old I had a skin test done in hospital and it showed strong reactions to pork, eggs, chocolate, and peanuts. To my surprise the migraines decreased significantly

when I avoided these things. Because I still had some symptoms, we decided to carry out thorough investigations as to what else I could be allergic to. First, a basic diet was compiled with the help of a dietitian. This consisted of potatoes, one type of vegetable, one type of bread (without additives or preservatives), butter, beef, peeled apples, and water. Everything went really well for a week, so I was allowed to extend the diet gradually, but I was told that I must not eat rice, cod, mushrooms, nor any foodstuff with a particular yellow colouring agent. After about 10 weeks of experimenting with various foods, I was able to choose from a selection of foodstuffs which didn't cause any allergic reactions. I'm glad I persevered. I'm particularly grateful to my parents and friends, because without their support and understanding I would never have stuck to the diet! The dietitian gave me a long list of foods to which I'm not hypersensitive. There's also a whole list of products I can't eat any more, but that's a sacrifice I'm willing to make for a life without migraines!'

3. The components which cause food allergy and food intolerance

Basically, any food component can cause food allergy or food intolerance in someone who is 'sensitive' to it. Common allergens include: cow's milk protein, chicken, egg yolk, fish, soya protein, some colouring agents (see Appendix I), preservatives and various metals which are present in food. Reactions are also often caused by bananas, old cheese, nuts, chocolate, wine, strawberries, shellfish, certain herbs and spices, fish, pork, and tomatoes.

An allergy to cow's milk protein is found in around 3-5% of infants, and these children tend to be generally irritable and cry a lot. They often suffer from diarrhoea, vomiting, respiratory difficulties and skin disorders, and the symptoms may appear a few minutes after the consumption of

Figure 5.10.1
© Daily Mail 28/12/93

Hidden peanuts threaten lives of children

by *Jenny Hope*, Medical Correspondent

... There have been four deaths this year from peanut allergy. Depending on the type of exposure, victims suffer symptoms ranging from swelling of the mouth and throat and puffy face to extreme anaphylactic shock which can trigger a fatal breathing crisis or heart attack.

The only effective way of stopping a severe reaction is an injection of adrenaline, which rapidly reverses the shock. It should usually be given within minutes. So, some sufferers are advised to always carry a shot with them.

Specialists fear people may now be overexposed to peanuts and peanut derived substances from an early age. Allergies are first formed when people become sensitised to an allergen when a substance is thought to be foreign by the body's immune response.

Allergic reactions then occur stronger and faster on second or subsequent exposures. With something like a peanut allergy, the immune system forms antibodies against a harmless food because it is misidentified as potentially harmful or foreign proteins.

Babies may become sensitised through exposure to baby milks and foods containing peanut oil (even some vitamin D preparations contain the oil) or perhaps because of peanuts eaten by breast-feeding mothers. Other experts believe peanuts in the pregnant woman's diet may set up the unborn baby for an allergy later in life.

Scientist Stan Bachelor's wife Brenda, who had a craving for peanut butter sandwiches while pregnant with their son Peter, now 12, believes that is where the boy's allergy originated.

"He was a toddler when he had his first attack, after eating a peanut butter sandwich," says Stan, of Billericay, Essex. "We went straight to our GP and he was glad we did – Peter could have died."

A study carried out by Dr David Hide, director of the clinical allergy research unit at St May's Hospital, Isle of Wight, suggests that one per cent of babies born there in 1989 have been sensitised to peanuts.

"It's a moot argument whether the sensitisation takes place before or after birth, though most children are probably sensitised afterwards. I think we would be better off reducing the exposure of both unborn babies and children to peanuts."

Dr Bill Frankland, consultant allergist at Guy's Hospital, London, is concerned that the presence of peanuts and peanut oils in a wide range of foods eaten by babies and toddlers may be a major factor in the apparent growth of the problem.

He points out that sometimes allergy victims do not react to the raw product. "Cooked peanuts cause the biggest problems, either in their original form, such as in peanut butter, or as peanut vegetable oil."

Dr Frankland believes that within five years there will be an effective way of shutting off peanut allergy reaction before it begins, using new vaccines being developed by scientists at Aston Science Park, Birmingham.

Preliminary trials of a vaccine designed to combat peanut allergy and hay fever start in January.

All-pervasive additive

PEANUTS are not actually nuts. They are members of the legume family, which includes beans, peas and lentils.

They are used extensively in Thai, Chinese and Indian cookery and are also found in some baby milks and other foods including chocolate bars, cakes, pies, biscuits and ice cream toppings.

In recent years, food manufacturers have seized upon peanuts as a novel additive for basic foods, too. There is now hardly anything that might not contain them, as any mother of an allergic child will testify.

They are often used as a cheap alternative to chopped almonds in biscuits and puddings.

Modern processing systems may also allow traces to contaminate foods that were never intended to contain peanuts.

the cow's milk or they may take several days to appear. The symptoms disappear, however, after the child stops taking cow's milk. Soya milk, supplemented with vitamins and minerals can be used as a substitute. If there is also an allergic reaction to the soya milk, special foods containing protein hydrolytes may be used. A diet which excludes cow's milk protein must be strictly adhered to because even traces of cow's milk protein can cause reactions. This allergy usually disappears by the time the child is 1–1½ years old.

Allergies to milk are common and, though symptomatic, are relatively harmless. The common presentation may be a rash (eczematoid). There are, however, increasing reports of rather more serious reactions to ingestion of foods such as peanuts and these can result in anaphylaxis (widespread vasodilation causing blood vessel collapse). This is potentially fatal (Figure 5.10.1).

4. Tracing the cause of food allergy or food intolerance

Sometimes the patient knows what he or she is allergic to, but diagnosing the allergy is usually a complicated matter. Skin tests and laboratory testing can help but the results are not one hundred per cent reliable.

In order to find out precisely which substances are causing an allergic reaction, a very basic diet called an elimination diet is drawn up. This requires the patient to eat for a few weeks only a narrow range of basic foods which are not suspected of causing the allergic reaction. These foods are often unprocessed and free of additives. If the symptoms disappear, it establishes what the patient is not allergic to. Then one additional food is tried and the reactions of the patient are carefully observed. If this does not cause any symptoms, other foods can be tested, one at a time, in the same manner. After a while a provocation test can be given, in which foods suspected of causing allergic reactions are reintroduced in the diet. If the symptoms reappear, a reliable diagnosis can then be made.

With the help of a dietitian and the Food Intolerance Databank based in Leatherhead, Surrey, an individual elimination diet can be designed. This databank provides extensive information about the composition of different foods, and it is possible, from the information they supply, to assemble a list of branded foods to which the patient will not be hypersensitive. The intention is to allow as much freedom of choice in the daily diet as possible.

Study activity

John is a year old and allergic to cow's milk protein. His typical daily diet is:
breakfast
–   1 slice of brown bread with margarine and marmalade
during the morning
–   1 glass of milk
lunch
–   2 slices of brown bread with margarine and cheese or luncheon meat
during the afternoon
–   1 glass of milk
–   1 piece of fruit
dinner
–   1 small portion of meat with a spoonful of gravy
–   1 serving of vegetables
–   1 potato
–   1 carton of yoghurt
    How do you think his diet should be modified?

5. Breast-feeding and hypersensitivity

Human milk has a unique composition adapted by nature to the infant's needs. It also contains immunity characteristics which protect the baby from infections and it has a protective effect for children who have a hereditary predisposition to hypersensitivity. In order to decrease the risk of the infant developing hypersensitivity it is often recommended that mothers breast-feed their babies for the first six months.

6. Summary

The symptoms associated with food allergy and food intolerance vary greatly between individuals, and each patient has a distinctive pattern of symptoms. These may affect the skin, the gastrointestinal tract, and the respiratory passages, and neuro-logical symptoms may also occur. It is usually difficult to establish an accurate diagnosis, but useful techniques include skin tests, laboratory tests, elimination diets, and provocation tests. The therapy consists of avoidance of the foods which cause allergic reactions and, while this may sound simple, the help of a dietitian is usually needed. The dietitian can help to compile an extensive list of products which will not affect the individual patient, and which will still be sufficient to constitute a nutritional and well-balanced diet.

11

Exploratory diets

1. Introduction

An exploratory diet is a tool used in making diagnoses. It lasts for only a short period, while the composition of the faeces, blood or urine is being investigated, and it involves the restriction or complete avoidance of certain foodstuffs because of the effect which they have on the investigation. Strict adherence to the diet is crucial to the success of the tests, and the patient and his or her family must be adequately informed. Even one divergence from the diet can corrupt the test results and require repetition of the entire procedure.

Two examples of exploratory diets are discussed in this chapter.

Learning outcomes

After studying this chapter, the student should be able to:
– explain the function of an exploratory diet, giving two examples;
– explain why it is important for a patient to be given adequate information about an exploratory diet.

2. Two examples of an exploratory diet

The haemoglobin-free diet
This diet is used to determine whether there is any haemorrhage in the gastro-intestinal tract. Foods which contain red blood cell pigments (haemoglobin) must therefore be avoided. These include all meats and chicken, and any products which are derived from them. Medication which might cause gastrointestinal haemorrhages (e.g. aspirin) is also avoided. After several days of the diet, the faecal matter is tested for the presence of blood components.

The constant fat intake diet
This diet is used to evaluate the digestion and absorption of fat by the body. The amount of fat the patient needs every day is carefully calculated, and it is precisely this amount that is given in the diet. This means that every food which contains fat must be carefully measured and the exact amount of fat calculated. After a time the faecal matter is tested. If the fat deposit is considerably higher than normal, meaning that the patient has steatorrhoea, or fatty diarrhoea, it may indicate disease of the pancreas or a disorder of the small intestine.

Exploratory diets usually last for anything up to a week. These diets differ between hospitals and depend on the particular type of research methods in use. If the diet is not fully adhered to, or if there are mistakes in its administration (which can occur even when the patient and his or her family have been given comprehensive instructions), it is very important that the doctor supervising the tests is informed. Otherwise, the wrong conclusions may be drawn from the results and this may have serious consequences.

3. Challenge diets

These diets are used to confirm the diagnosis of sensitivity to various substances. One example is the glucose tolerance test where a challenge of glucose is used to provoke elevation of blood glucose concentration. A steep rise and slow fall in blood glucose is diagnostic of diabetes mellitus. Other examples include challenges of lactose to determine lactose intolerance, and a challenge of gluten to assist in the diagnosis of coeliac disease.

4. Summary

Exploratory and challenge diets are used as tools for making a diagnosis. The haemoglobin-free diet and the constant fat intake diet were discussed, and both of these diets require that certain foodstuffs be avoided or restricted for a short period of time, to enable tests on faecal matter to be carried out free from extraneous influence. It is crucial that the diet is strictly followed, and that the patient and the people in close contact with him are given adequate information, as even one small divergence from the diet can render the test results invalid.

12

Diet and mental health

1. Introduction

In general, there is no reason why the diet of someone who is mentally ill should differ from an average healthy diet, but there is a wide variety of potential problems with varying degrees of seriousness. Even relatively trivial problems, if they recur daily, can lead to both the health care workers and the patients being caught up in a tense atmosphere of concern and anxiety.

This chapter deals with the causes of some common eating and drinking problems among the mentally ill, and offers some possible solutions.

Learning outcomes

After studying this chapter the student should be able to:
– understand some of the factors which can cause eating and drinking problems among the mentally ill;
– suggest possible solutions to these problems.

2. The causes of eating and drinking problems among the mentally ill

While the recommendations for a normal healthy diet (see Chapter 2 of Module 2) apply equally to the mentally ill, there are many factors which can influence the eating and drinking patterns of these patients and which must therefore be considered. Such factors range from impatience and tension on the part of the health care workers to the seriousness and nature of the patient's mental impairment. People who are mentally ill may also have related disorders such as motor dysfunction, sensory dysfunction, epilepsy, contact dysfunction and behavioural disorders and, in order to gain insight into the causes of their eating and drinking disorders, the following factors should be considered.

a. Factors stemming from the individual
There are several possible intrinsic causes of eating problems: problems with reflexes in the mouth, oral sensitivity, and tension in the facial muscles used when eating; in some babies, the sucking reflexes are absent; oral reflexes can be too easily stimulated, leading to gagging and food entering the windpipe; the mouth area is often oversensitive, causing an exaggerated reaction when the inside of the mouth is touched.

Conversely, there can be a lack of sensitivity in the mouth area, causing other eating and drinking problems. If there is too little or too much tension in the mouth muscles, drinking and taking food from a spoon become impossible. Biting and chewing are often impossible, and swallowing may be prevented by the tongue pushing food back out of the mouth.

The appetite can also be depressed for various reasons, some of which have been discussed in Chapter 3 of this module.

People who are mentally ill often have an abnormally slow rate of growth, so their diet should be adapted to them as individuals rather than to their age group. It is quite possible for a child of two to have the height and weight of a child of one, and his or her nutritional requirements will therefore be those of a one-year-old.

If a person is relatively immobile and takes very little physical exercise, the energy requirement will be low and the risk of obesity increases. This is also true if there is unrestricted eating behaviour. In contrast, people who suffer from spasms have an increased energy requirement.

Some people cannot properly express the fact that they are thirsty, and in such cases it is important that health care workers pay close attention to the fluid intake of such patients and maintain a fluid chart, if necessary.

With the use of certain types of medication, there may be an increased need for vitamins and minerals (see Chapter 3 of this module). Regular vomiting and regurgitation of food can also pose a problem in that this increases the risk of malnutrition. In addition, constipation is a common complaint caused by the use of certain medicines, the lack of physical activity, insufficient fluid intake, a lack of dietary fibre and a slow metabolism.

b. External factors

A chaotic atmosphere during meal times or impatience on the part of health care workers can give rise to anxiety in people who are mentally ill and result in a refusal to eat. Excessive noise in the room can cause a shock reaction and result in increased muscle tension which impedes eating and drinking.

Posture can also cause problems. For example, if the head of a mentally ill child is held too far back, the child will not have the opportunity to participate actively in the eating process, and the food may dribble out of the mouth.

Other factors which may cause disturbance and discomfort include inadequately adapted utensils, a table laid in a disorganised manner, pressure on cheeks or jaws as the health care worker holds the patient's face still to facilitate feeding, overeating of sweets between meals and irregularity of meal times.

3. Possible solutions

In a hospital or residential care environment, if and when these problems occur, solutions must be found. This is usually effected by teamwork, and may involve parents, the doctor, the speech therapist, the dietitian, and nursing staff.

If the problems are intrinsic ones concerning an individual patient, the following points may contribute to their solution:
–   If there is a risk of choking, thicker fluids cause fewer problems than thinner ones like coffee, tea, milk, and fruit juices. Liquid can be taken in the form of porridge, yoghurt, and fluids which contain binding agents. Thinner drinks can be artificially thickened. Finely mashed fruit is also a healthful source of liquid;
–   A speech therapist may be able to help develop and improve the motor functioning of the mouth when eating and drinking, to make biting, chewing, drinking and swallowing easier for the patient;
–   Make the hole in the rubber nipple of bottles bigger for children who have difficulty sucking;
–   If a cup is used for drinking, it is best to use one with a slightly curved rim. When the cup is tilted so that the fluid level reaches the lips, the patient will be able to take a sip himself. Swallowing is stimulated by the pressure on the bottom of the mouth;
–   It is best not to use a cup with a spout as this may provoke inappropriate

mouth activities such as biting and abnormal tongue movement;
- Ensure that appropriate utensils are used for eating, and that they are neither too wide nor too long. Place the food on the front part of the spoon, place the spoon in the mouth straight and level, and press the spoon firmly down on the tongue. This will prevent the tongue coming forward. Keep the mouth closed until the food has been swallowed;
- If constipation occurs, ensure that intake of fluid and dietary fibre is sufficient;
- Providing semi-solid food, and providing distractions immediately after meals can help to prevent regular vomiting and regurgitation;
- Try to encourage the patient to follow a healthy diet which is adapted to his individual needs. Ensure that meal times are regular, and limit the intake of sweets between meals;
- If serious chewing and swallowing problems prevent consumption of normal food, tube feeding may be used. A dietitian can help with selecting the type, volume, and composition of the tube-feed.

If the eating problems are caused by external factors, the following suggestions may help:
- Ensure that there is a calm, relaxed atmosphere at the table, and be patient with anyone who is having difficulties;
- Place the plate and cup on the table directly in front of the patient so that he or she can see where the food is coming from. Lay the table in a neat, organised manner;
- Ensure that the patient is sitting with a good posture and do not hold the food or drink so high that the patient has to lean back;
- Take the patient's tastes and preferences into account. In response to a depressed appetite, try the recommendations given in Chapter 3 of this module;
- Do not force patients to eat. Refusal of food may be a sign that the patient is full, that the food does not taste very appetising or that the patient is tired or out of sorts.

Study activity 1

What problems can arise as a result of a lack of sensitivity in the mouth area?

Study activity 2

Norman is 7 years old and mentally ill. He suffers from impaired muscular function and is epileptic. He tires easily and is susceptible to infection. His body weight has remained constant over the past year, despite his having grown taller. He can eat without help, but it requires a lot of effort. Which of the following foods do you think are suitable for Norman? Which do you think he should avoid? Give reasons for your answers.
Semi-skimmed milk, full fat milk, eggs, peas, soft drinks, diluted orange squash, milk shakes, chocolate, pieces of cheese, nuts, crisps, low fat margarine, fresh fruit, white bread, wholemeal bread, braising steak, minced beef, water.

4. Summary

As a general rule, the normal recommendations for a healthy diet also apply to people who are mentally ill. However, a wide variety of eating and drinking problems can occur. Some of these may be caused by the extent and nature of the handicap and its related disorders, but external factors can also play a role. Possible solutions for some common eating and drinking problems were suggested. It is essential that health care workers maintain a high level of attention and patience when dealing with people who are mentally ill.

Diet and phenylketonuria (PKU)

1. Introduction

Since the 1960s, all newborn children in the UK are screened for phenylketonuria (a metabolic disorder) by means of the Guthrie test. This screening takes place 6-10 days after birth. If the condition is diagnosed, the child will be referred to a teaching hospital for treatment. Early treatment and a strict diet can prevent serious complications. Phenylketonuria occurs in 1 out of every 5,000-10,000 live births.

Learning outcomes

After studying this chapter the student should be able to:
- explain in his or her own words what phenylketonuria is;
- explain the objective of the diet used in treating phenylketonuria;
- give a brief description of a phenylalanine-restricted diet and say why this diet has such drastic implications for the patient and his or her family and friends;
- list the supplements which are necessary to make this a balanced diet.

2. What is phenylketonuria?

Phenylketonuria is a genetic metabolic disorder in which the enzyme phenylalanine hydroxylase is either deficient or absent. As a result, the amino acid phenylalanine, which is absorbed through food, is not converted or is insufficiently converted to tyrosine (which is also an amino acid). Consequently, phenylalanine accumulates in the blood and, if untreated, the condition can lead to irreparable brain damage, and mental retardation. Early treatment can prevent this deterioration.

3. How is phenylketonuria treated?

The treatment for phenylketonuria consists of a phenylalanine-restricted diet.

Phenylalanine is an essential amino acid found in all proteins. The amount of phenylalanine which may be ingested depends on the patient's age and body weight, and the level of phenylalanine in the patient's blood.

Being an essential amino acid, phenylketonuria is vital for growth and development and, in order to obtain the optimum benefit from the restricted amount allowed in food, it is best to extend the intake over the course of the day. In addition, normal intake of the other amino acids must be maintained for use in the structure and maintenance of the body cells. In practice this means that:
- specially prepared low protein bread must be substituted for ordinary bread;

- foods which contain protein, such as milk, can only be taken in limited quantities. In general, meat, fish, eggs, and chicken are avoided;
- a low phenylalanine amino acid preparation (a mixture of amino acids, vitamins, and minerals in powder form) must be used to supplement the deficient diet. It is the patient's principal protein source. It can be served in a liquid or taken by spoon and mixed to a paste. It does not taste good, but if an individual has been taking it since birth this should not pose a problem.

4. Duration of treatment

The general opinion is that the phenylalanine-restricted diet should be followed for as long as possible. There is a risk that if a person diverges from the diet too early damage to the central nervous system could still occur.

It is also necessary for a pregnant PKU patient to follow the diet as otherwise there is a risk that her child will be born with congenital disorders. When coming off the diet, the intake of foods which contain protein is gradually increased. Protein intake should still be restricted, although not as severely.

Study activity

a. Name two foods which do not contain protein and are thus suitable for mixing with a low phenylalanine amino acid preparation.
b. Discuss the possible social consequences for the family of a child who has phenylketonuria.

5. Summary

Phenylketonuria is one of the most well-known amino acid metabolic disorders. Every newborn child is screened for this disease. It can be treated but it must be detected at an early stage, and the diet strictly followed.

Final Test for Module 5

Instructions

This section consists of 114 statements. Each one may be correct or incorrect. The answer required is either YES or NO. In your assessment of whether the statement is correct or incorrect, you may only base your answer on the information given. The questions are arranged in groups, in the order that the related topics occurred in the text.

After ensuring that all the questions have been answered, check the answers yourself in the back of the book.

1. A prescribed diet differs from an ordinary balanced diet for medical reasons, and it is exactly the same no matter for whom it is prescribed.
2. Dietary advice is given by a dietitian. It consists of practical dietary information and is adapted to the preferences of the patient as much as possible.
3. A vegetarian diet is one example of a nutrient-restricted diet.
4. If a prescribed diet is adapted to the tastes and preferences of a patient, it is easier for the patient to maintain the diet.
5. If a patient is adequately informed about his prescribed diet, he will be able to deal with the diet more easily and independently.
6. Hypoglycaemia can occur in people with diabetes if they have not eaten for a while, or if they have eaten too little.
7. A diabetic cannot take wholemeal biscuits or fruit loaf freely.

8. A diabetic is usually allowed a glass of spirits or wine.
9. People with diabetes must always weigh any foods which contain carbohydrates.
10. Sorbitol provides as much energy as ordinary sugar.
11. Special products for diabetics, such as sugar-free biscuits or chocolate, can be consumed without restriction in a low energy diabetic diet.
12. A diabetic may participate in sports activities.
13. It is possible for a diabetic to eat in a restaurant.
14. There is a relationship between obesity and diabetes type II.
15. A diabetic can drink as much unsweetened fruit juice as he or she wants.
16. If a type II diabetic who is obese attains a normal body weight, the diabetic medication can be decreased.
17. In hypoglycaemia the blood glucose level is too low.
18. It is better for a diabetic to have an orange than a glass of unsweetened orange juice.
19. It is recommended that a diabetic eat three times a day rather than six times a day.
20. Type I diabetes is usually treated with insulin and a prescribed diet.
21. Having a few pieces of cheese with an alcoholic drink can prevent hypoglycaemia in a diabetic.
22. The most important basic principle of a diabetic diet is ensuring that the

supply of carbohydrates in the meals is distributed evenly over the day.

23. In principle, people with diabetes can take sugar if the meal also contains protein, fat or dietary fibre, and if the amount of carbohydrates in the meal corresponds with that in the prescribed diet.

24. When malnutrition is present a person is more susceptible to infection and it takes longer for wounds to heal.

25. It is better for people with a depressed appetite to eat three times a day than to eat six small meals over the course of the day.

26. People with a poor appetite should not have a lot of fat in their diet as fat slows down digestion.

27. Whipped cream in drinks and on desserts is recommended for people with a depressed appetite.

28. Fats which are not emulsified (such as those in fatty meat and gravy) are easier and quicker to digest than the fats in full fat milk and whipped cream.

29. For someone who has poor nutritional status, extra protein in the diet will only be of use if the diet also contains sufficient energy.

30. Foods suitable for an energy-enriched and protein-enriched diet include full fat milk, cheese, cream and egg.

31. Although obesity is far more prevalent in our affluent society than malnutrition, the latter is the main cause for concern.

32. A number of people in hospitals and nursing homes are in a more or less serious state of malnutrition.

33. Weight loss, muscular weakness, listlessness, loose skin, and paleness of the skin and of the mucous membranes can all indicate poor nutritional status.

34. It is best to take iron preparations along with a glass of milk.

35. It is recommended that patients with a low potassium level in the blood take extra fruit or fruit juice.

36. Malnourished people are always thin.

37. If you have a hiatus hernia, it is better to eat three times a day rather than eat six small meals a day.

38. It is better for people with a hiatus hernia not to go to sleep or lie down directly after a meal.

39. A special prescribed diet is necessary for a person with a peptic ulcer.

40. One important recommendation for people with peptic ulcers is that they should try to have their meals in peaceful and quiet surroundings.

41. Fizzy drinks should be avoided if you have diarrhoea.

42. It would be best for people with peptic ulcers to avoid the foods which cause problems, but to try them again after a suitable time lapse.

43. If you experience gastric problems as the result of an ulcer, it is better to eat small meals more often than to eat three full meals a day.

44. People whose stomach has been made smaller by surgery are advised to drink a lot with their meals.

45. A patient on a lactose-free diet may not have milk or yoghurt.

46. Suitable drinks for people suffering from diarrhoea include water, apple juice, tea, grape juice and thin soup with a low fat content.

47. Ordinary bread can be eaten in a gluten-free diet.

48. People with a colostomy need a special prescribed diet.

49. People with a colostomy should make sure that they chew food thoroughly.

50. People with a colostomy are more likely to have thin, watery stools than people with an ileostomy.

51. If constipation is persistent, the risk of haemorrhoids increases.

52. There is no point in maintaining an intake rich in dietary fibre if you do not take enough fluids.

53. Examples of products rich in dietary fibre include: wholemeal bread, apples, meat, pulses, and peanut butter.

54. Yoghurt and buttermilk can have a

slight laxative effect.

55. People with diverticulosis are advised to eat white bread, rice, and crackers.

56. Patients with pancreatic disorders generally benefit from a low fat, healthy diet without alcohol.

57. For people with hepatitis or pancreatitis, several small meals taken throughout the course of the day are usually easier to deal with than three large meals.

58. If a person has gallstones, he or she will always suffer symptoms from them.

59. No one who suffers colic attacks as a result of gallstones may have egg yolk, coffee, or foods rich in fat.

60. Obese people run a greater risk of developing gallstones.

61. Eating something before going to sleep can contribute to the prevention of stone formation in the gall bladder.

62. A meal consisting of lean pork, boiled potatoes and runner beans with lean gravy would be suitable for anyone with chronic pancreatitis and diarrhoea.

63. Minced food is an example of food with an altered consistency.

64. Where chewing or swallowing problems persist, minced or liquid food might be necessary to prevent malnutrition.

65. Brown bread without the crust and a soft sandwich spread can be components of a diet based on minced foods.

66. A diet based on minced foods is usually rich in dietary fibre.

67. In a diet based on minced foods, it is best to mix together the minced meat, vegetables, and mashed potatoes.

68. One area for attention in the care of patients with swallowing problems is the prevention of dehydration.

69. Inadequate hygiene when using a tube feed can cause diarrhoea in a patient.

70. You never need to rinse the tubes used for tube feeding.

71. Monomer food is pre-digested food and results in a reduced amount of faeces.

72. If a patient is being fed by a tube feed,

he or she can never eat or drink any additional nutriments.

73. If you are suffering from stomatitis (inflammation of the mucous membranes of the mouth), drinking camomile tea can alleviate the pain.

74. Risk factors for heart and arterial disease include a high cholesterol level in the blood and hypertension.

75. A high cholesterol level in the blood can be reduced by a diet rich in saturated fats.

76. Sodium is a mineral which is not essential to our body.

77. Oedema can be alleviated by following a low sodium diet.

78. Ready-made soups and sauces usually contain a lot of salt.

79. In a low sodium diet, sea salt can be used as a substitute for ordinary table salt.

80. Low sodium bread dries out more quickly than ordinary bread.

81. In a diet in which sodium is only slightly restricted, special low salt milk must be used.

82. If a patient is taking diuretics (but not potassium-sparing diuretics), it is recommended that he or she eat extra fruit, vegetables or potatoes.

83. A patient who has had a CVA often does not drink enough.

84. Oil, nuts, and diet margarine can raise the cholesterol level in the blood.

85. Salt alternatives can often be used in a low sodium diet as a substitute for ordinary salt.

86. It is recommended that people with hypertension maintain a normal body weight.

87. A diet in which sodium is only slightly restricted (NAS) differs from a normal diet in only one respect: food should not be salted at the table.

88. Patients with impaired kidney function frequently complain of nausea and often have a depressed appetite.

89. A patient with impaired kidney function will usually have fewer symptoms if he or she reduces the amount of

protein in the diet.

90. In cases of renal disorder, the diet should contain few carbohydrates or fats in order to prevent the body proteins from being broken down.

91. Foods high in protein include margarine, fruit, and vegetables.

92. A patient on a low protein diet may never have milk.

93. Special low protein toast or crackers can usually be eaten without restriction in a low protein diet.

94. A patient with impaired kidney function and a poor appetite will benefit from two large meals a day.

95. The risk of kidney stones is decreased by drinking a lot.

96. If a patient with cancer has good nutritional status, he or she will usually be better equipped to cope with the various forms of treatment.

97. Patients with cancer usually have a good appetite.

98. There is no point in trying to improve a patient's nutritional status at an early stage of cancer.

99. When a sore throat is caused by an infection of the mucous membrane, it is better to drink orange juice than milk.

100. A diet high in energy and protein is often advised for cancer patients.

101. Buttermilk and yoghurt stimulate production of mucus more than milk does.

102. Insufficient fluid intake while undergoing radiotherapy or chemotherapy can promote feelings of nausea.

103. The Bristol Diet contains primarily products without chemical additives.

104. Treatment with chemotherapy or radiotherapy can cause insufficient production of saliva, a loss of or a change in the sense of taste, nausea and vomiting.

105. A patient who maintains a healthy diet will feel better and suffer less from fatigue and listlessness.

106. Eczema, stomachache, chronic colds, asthma, and migraines are all symptoms which can indicate allergic reactions to food.

107. Certain colouring agents and preservatives can cause food allergies or food intolerance in people who are hypersensitive to them.

108. It is estimated that 1 in 50 infants is hypersensitive to cow's milk protein.

109. By using an elimination diet, it is possible to determine to which foods a person is allergic.

110. The objective of an exploratory diet is to test the patient's sense of taste.

111. A single divergence from the prescribed foods could cause an exploratory diet to fail.

112. One example of an exploratory diet is the constant fat intake diet.

113. A low phenylalanine diet must be followed by people suffering from phenylketonuria.

114. Brain damage resulting from PKU can be prevented by restricting the amount of phenylalanine, within a few weeks of birth, to the minimum needed for growth.

References and further reading

Ball M and Mann J, (1988) *Lipids and Heart Disease: A Practical Approach.* Oxford University Press, Oxford.

Barnes K E, (1990) An examination of nurses' feelings about patients with specific feeding needs. *Journal of Advanced Nursing,* 15, (6), 703-711.

Bennett S E et al, (1983) Low protein diets in uraemia. *British Medical Journal,* 287, 1344-1345.

Briony T (ed), (1994) *Manual of Dietetic Practice.* 2nd ed. Blackwell Scientific Publications,.Oxford.

British Nutrition Foundation Briefing Paper No. 26, (1992) *Coronary Heart Disease, The Wider Perspective.* British Nutrition Foundation, London.

Brostoff J and Challacombe S, (1987) *Food Allergy and Intolerance.* Bailliere Tindall, London.

Cann P A et al, (1984) What is the benefit of coarse wheat bran in patients with irritable bowel syndrome? *Gut.* 24, 168-173.

Cataldo C, De Bruyne L and Whitney E, (1992) *Nutrition and Diet Therapy.*3rd ed. West Publishing Co., New York.

The Coeliac Society, *The Coeliac Handbook.* The Coeliac Society, High Wycombe.

Day J L et al, (1992) *Living with Non-Insulin Dependant Diabetes.* 2nd ed. Medikos, Crowborough.

Holmes S, (1991) Nutrition and the surgical patient. *Nursing Times,* 86 (8), 68-72.

Nutrition Sub-Committee, British Diabetic Association, (1991) *Dietary Recommendation for People with Diabetes: An Update for the 1990s.* British Diabetic Association, London.

Scottish Office Home and Health Department, (1993) *The Scottish Diet: Report of a Working Party for the Chief Medical Officer of Health for Scotland.* HMSO, Edinburgh.

Sherlock S, (1989) *Diseases of the Liver and Biliary System.* 6th ed. Blackwell Scientific Publications, Oxford.

Shireff A, (1990) Pre-operative nutritional assessment. *Nursing Times,* 86 ,(8), 68-72

Sonsken P et al, (1991) *Diabetes at your Fingertips.* Class Publishing, London.

Torrance C (1991), Pre-operative nutrition, fasting and the surgical patient. *Surgical Nurse,* 5, (4), 5-8.

Watkins P J, Drury P L and Taylor K W (1990) *Diabetes and its Management.* Blackwell Scientific Publications, London.

Whitney and Rolfes S, (1993) *Understanding Nutrition.* 6th ed. West Publishing Company, New York.

Workman E et al, (1984) *The Allergy Diet – How to Overcome Food Intolerance.* Martin Dunitz, London.

Answers to final test for Module 1

1. no	4. no	7. yes	10. yes
2. yes	5. no	8. no	11. no
3. yes	6. yes	9. yes	12. no

Answers to final test for Module 2

1. yes	18. yes	35. yes	52. yes	69. yes	86. no
2. no	19. no	36. yes	53. yes	70. yes	87. no
3. yes	20. yes	37. yes	54. no	71. no	88. yes
4. no	21. yes	38. no	55. no	72. no	89. yes
5. yes	22. no	39. yes	56. yes	73. yes	90. yes
6. yes	23. yes	40. yes	57. no	74. no	
7. no	24. yes	41. yes	58. yes	75. yes	
8. yes	25. yes	42. yes	59. yes	76. no	
9. yes	26. yes	43. no	60. yes	77. yes	
10. no	27. yes	44. yes	61. no	78. yes	
11. yes	28. yes	45. no	62 yes	79. yes	
12. yes	29. no	46. no	63. no	80. no	
13. yes	30. yes	47. yes	64. no	81. yes	
14. no	31. yes	48. no	65. yes	82. yes	
15. no	32. yes	49. no	66. yes	83. yes	
16. no	33. no	50. no	67. no	84. yes	
17. no	34. yes	51. no	68. yes	85. yes	

Answers to final test for Module 3

1. no	11. no	21. no	31. no	41. no
2. yes	12. yes	22. yes	32. no	42. yes
3. no	13. yes	23. no	33. yes	43. no
4. yes	14. no	24. no	34. yes	44. no
5. no	15. yes	25. no	35. no	45. yes
6. yes	16. yes	26. no	36. yes	46. no
7. yes	17. no	27. yes	37. yes	47. yes
8. no	18. no	28. yes	38. yes	48. no
9. no	19. yes	29. no	39. yes	49. yes
10. yes	20. yes	30. no	40. no	50. no

Answers to final test for Module 4

1. no	6. yes	11. yes	16. yes	21. yes
2. yes	7. yes	12. yes	17. yes	22. no
3. yes	8. yes	13. yes	18. yes	
4. no	9. no	14. no	19. yes	
5. yes	10. no	15. no	20. no	

Answers to final test for Module 5

1. no	21. no	41. no	61. yes	81. no	101. no
2. yes	22. yes	42. yes	62. yes	82. yes	102. yes
3. no	23. yes	43. yes	63. yes	83. yes	103. yes
4. yes	24. yes	44. no	64. yes	84. yes	104. yes
5. yes	25. no	45. yes	65. yes	85. yes	105. yes
6. yes	26. yes	46. yes	66. no	86. yes	106. yes
7. yes	27. no	47. no	67. no	87. no	107. yes
8. yes	28. no	48. no	68. yes	88. yes	108. yes
9. no	29. yes	49. yes	69. yes	89. yes	109. yes
10. yes	30. yes	50. no	70. no	90. no	110. no
11. no	31. yes	51. yes	71. yes	91. no	111. yes
12. yes	32. yes	52. yes	72. no	92. no	112. yes
13. yes	33. yes	53. no	73. yes	93. yes	113. no
14. yes	34. no	54. yes	74. yes	94. no	114. yes
15. no	35. yes	55. no	75. no	95. yes	
16. yes	36. no	56. yes	76. no	96. yes	
17. yes	37. no	57. yes	77. yes	97. no	
18. yes	38. yes	58. no	78. yes	98. no	
19. no	39. no	59. no	79. no	99. no	
20. yes	40. yes	60. yes	80. yes	100. yes	

Appendix 1 List of food additives

Additives with the prefix E (European) have been accepted as safe throughout the European Union. Numbers without the E prefix have been accepted as safe within the United Kingdom while awaiting approval by the European Union,

COLOURING

Colour is lost in food processing and this can be replaced artificially to give back the original colour, thus making the food look more 'natural' and appetising. There are appproximately 20 artificial colours permitted with others coming from natural sources. The colours are normally in the E100 series.

E100	Curcumin
E101	Ribloflavin or Lactoflavin
101 (a)	Riboflavin-5'-Phosphate
E102	Tartrazine
E104	Quinoline Yellow
E110	Sunset Yellow
E120	Conchineal
E122	Carmoisine
E123	Amaranth
E124	Ponceau 4R
E127	Erythrosine
128	Red 2G
E132	Indigo Carmine
133	Brilliant Blue
E140	Chlorophyll
E141	Copper complex of Chlorophyll
E142	Green S
E150	Caramel
E151	Black PN
E153	Carbon Black (Vegetable Carbon)
154	Brown FK
155	Chocolate Brown HT

E160 (a-f)	Carotenoids and Derivatives
E161 (a-g)	Xanthophylls
E162	Betanin (Beetroot Red)
E163	Anthocyanins
	- Paprika Extract
	- Turmeric
	- Saffron
	- Crocin
	- Sandalwood

PRESERVATIVES

Preservatives protect food against growth of microbes which makes food deteriorate. They also help to increase storage life and are found mostly in the E200 section.

E200	Sorbic acid
E201	Sodium sorbate
E202	Potassium sorbate
E203	Calcium sorbate
E210	Benzoic acid
E211	Sodium benzoate
E212	Potassium benzoate
E213	Calcium benzoate
E214 –219	Hydroxybenzoate Salts
E220	Sulphur dioxide
E221	Sodium sulphite
E222	Sodium hydrogen sulphite/ bisulphite
E223	Sodium metabisulphite
E224	Potassium metabisulphite
E226	Calcium sulphite
E227	Calcium hydrogen sulphite

E230	Biphenyl
234	Nisin
E249	Potassium nitrite
E250	Sodium nitrite
E251	Sodium nitrate
E252	Potassium nitrate
E280	Propionic acid
E281	Sodium propionate
E282	Calcum propionate
E283	Potassium propionate

ANTIOXIDANTS

These prevent fatty food going rancid and help to stop fruit browning. They are generally in the E300 series.

E300	L-ascorbic acid (Vitamin C)
E301	Sodium L-ascorbate
E302	Calcium L-ascorbate
E304	Ascorbyl palmitate
E306	Tocopherols (Vitamin E)
E307	Alpha-tocopherol
E308	Gamma-tocopherol
E309	Delta-tocopherol
E310	Propyl gallate
E311	Octyl gallate
E312	Dodecyl gallate
E320	Butylated hydroxyanisole (BHA)
E330	Citric acid
E331	Sodium citrate
E332	Mono- or Tri-potassium citrate
E333	Mono-di- or Tri-calcium citrate

EMULSIFIERS AND STABILISERS

These help substances, such as oil and water, to blend easily. They also help to give some foods a smooth consistency without separating once they have been blended and also help to prevent baked foods from going stale.

E222	Lecithins
E400	Alginic acid
E401	Sodium alginate
E404	Calcium alginate
E406	Agar
E407	Carrageenan
E410	Locust bean (carob) gum
E412	Guar (cluster bean) gum
E413	Tragacanth
E414	Acacia (gum arabic)
E415	Xanthan gum
E440 (i)	Pectin
E440 (ii)	Amidated pectin
E450	Sodium & potassium phosphate salts
E471	Mono- & di-glycerides of fatty acids
E472	Substances prepared from E471
E475	Polyglycerol esters of fatty acids

FLAVOUR ENHANCERS

Flavour enhancers are added in small amounts to restore flavour lost in cooking.

620	L-glutamic acid
621	Monosodium glutamate (MSG)
627	Sodium guanylate
631	Sodium inosinate
635	Sodium 5'-ribonucleotide

SWEETENERS

These are very sweet substances with very low calorie value and they are usually used in soft drinks and confectionery

E420	Sorbitol
	Sorbitol syrup
	Thaumatin
E421	Mannitol
	Saccharin

OTHERS

Raising Agents
Anti-caking Agents
Acids
Flour Improvers
Thickening Agents
Nutrients

Appendix 2

Diabetes mellitus: carbohydrate exchange list

10 grams (g) carbohydrate = 1 exchange
One tablespoon (level) = 2 dessert spoons (level)
OR 15 ml standard level spoon

Each of the following is 1 exchange
Underlined items are foods high in dietary fibre content

BREAD

Wholemeal or white	$1/2$ large thick slice/1 small slice
Rolls, Baps	$1/2$ roll
Wholemeal roll	$1/2$ roll
Croissants	$1/2$ croissant
Butteries	
(Aberdeen rolls)	$1/2$ roll
Crumpets	1 small
Scones	$1/2$ large/1 small
Scotch pancake	$1/2$
Pitta bread	$1/3$ bread
Chapati	$1/2$ medium
Nan	$1/4$ bread

BREAKFAST CEREAL

All Bran, Bran Flakes	5 tablespoons
Cornflakes	5 tablespoons
Weetaflakes	4 tablespoons
Weetabix, Shredded Wheat	1 biscuit
Porridge, (cooked)	7 tablespoons
Rice Krispies, Special K	6 tablespoons
Muesli unsweetened	5 tablespoons
Bran Buds	3 tablespoons

RICE AND PASTA

Rice brown or white (cooked)	3 tablespoons/ 35g
Spaghetti wholemeal (uncooked)	20 short/10 long strands
Spaghetti white (uncooked)	20 short/10 long strands
Pasta white (cooked) eg. macaroni, noodles	3 tablespoons/ 40g
Pasta wholemeal (cooked)	3 tablespoons.45g
Ravioli tinned	$1/3$ small tin
Spaghetti tinned	$1/3$ small tin

FLOUR

Wholemeal/ wholewheat	$1^1/2$ tablespoons/ 15g

White plain/ self raising	1 tablespoon/15g

BISCUITS

Digestive, bran biscuits	1 large/2 small
Crispbread (wholewheat, rye)	2
Crackers plain or wholewheat	2
Plain, Rich Tea	2
Oatcakes	1 large/2 small
Matzos	2 small
Water biscuits	2

VEGETABLES

Most vegetables have such a low content of carbohydrate that they need not be counted in the diet if taken in normal portions. However, the following must be counted:-

Beans, baked in tomato sauce	5 tablespoons
Beans - dried, uncooked	2 tablespoons
Lentils - dried	2 tablespoons
Sweetcorn - canned or frozen	5 tablespoons
Corn on the cob	1/2 cob

POTATOES

Boiled	1 small (egg sized)
Jacket	1 medium (Egg size)
Chips	5 average
Crisps	1 small packet (25g)
Roast	1 small (egg sized)
Mashed	1 scoop

FRUIT

As with vegetables some fruits are low in carbohydrate and need not be counted if taken in normal quanties but the following should be counted:

Apple eating with skin	1 medium
cooking	1 medium
stewed without sugar	6 tablespoons

Apricots fresh or dried	4 medium
Banana	1 small
Cherries, fresh	15
Dates fresh	3 medium
dried	3 small
Dried fruit eg. raisin, currants, sultanas	1 1/2 tablespoons
Figs fresh or dried	1 large/2 small
Grapes	10 large
Greengages	3
Guavas fresh	1
Kiwi	2
Mango fresh	1/3 large
Nectarine fresh	1 medium
Orange	1 large
Paw-paw	1/4
Peach fresh	1 medium
Pear, eating with skin	1 medium
Pineapple fresh	1 thick slick
tinned in natural juice	2 rings
Plums dessert fresh	2 large/4 small
Prunes dried	3 medium
Satsumas, tangerines	2

FRUIT JUICE

Unsweetened fruit juice	1 small glass/ 100ml
Tomato juice	250ml

NUTS

Peanuts	100g
Mixed nuts and raisins	1 small packet/ 30g

MILK

Whole, semi-skimmed, skimmed	1 glass (200ml/1/3 pint)
Dried - skimmed/whole	4 tablespoons
Yoghurt -natural, fruit (diet)	1 small carton
fruit-sweetened	1/2 small carton

Milk pudding (Without sugar) 3 tablespoons

*Always add artificial sweetener <u>after</u>
cooking.

MISCELLANEOUS

Soup, thick, all types	1 ladle/150ml
Fish fingers - grilled	2
Pizza	$^1/_2$ snack size
Sausages - grilled	2 average/1 slice
Sausage roll	1 very small
White/black pudding	2 slices
Haggis - boiled	4 tablespoons
Spring roll (pancake roll)	1
Scotch pie with meat filling	$^1/_3$
Ice cream	1 scoop
Jelly (ready to eat)	3 tablespoons
Ovaltine/Bournvita/ Drinking Chocolate	3 teaspoons

Appendix 3
Useful addresses

Action Against Allergy, 43 The Downs, London SW20 8HS,

Association of Breastfeeding Mothers, 26 Hearnshaw Close, London SE26 4TH. Tel 081-778 4769.

BACUP (British Association for Cancer United Patients and their families and friends), 121/123 Charterhouse Street, London EC1M 6AA.
Tel Cancer Information Service 071-608 1661.

British Diebetic Association, 10 Queen Anne Street, London W1M 0BD.
Tel 071-323 1531; Fax 071-637 3644.

British Dietetic Association, 7th Floor, Elizabeth House, 22 Suffolk Street, Queensway, Birmingham B1 1LS.
Tel 021-643 5483,

British Geriatric Society, 1 St Andrew's Place, Regents Park, London NW1 4LB.

British Heart Foundation, 14 Fitzhardinge Street, London W1H 4DH, Tel 071-935 0185,

British Nutrition Foundation, High Holborn House, 52-54 High Holborn,London WC1V 6RU.
Tel 071-404 6504; Fax 071-404 6747.

CancerLink, 46 Pentonville Road, London N1, Tel 071-833 2451.

Coeliac Society, PO Box 220, High Wycombe, Bucks HP11 2HY.
Tel 0494 437278,

Coronary Prevention Group, 102 Gloucester Place, London W1H 3DA.
Tel 071-935 2889.

Department of Agriculture and Fisheries for Scotland, Chesser House, 500 Gorgie Road, Edinburgh EH11 3AW.

Department of Health, Nutrition Unit, Wellington House, 133-155 Waterloo Road, London SE1 8UG.
Tel 071-972 2000.

Eating Disorders Association, Sackville Place, 44 Magdalen Street, Norwich, Norfolk. Tel 0603 621414.

Family Heart Association, Wesley House, 7 High Street, Kidlington, Oxford OX5 2DH. Tel 08675 70292.

The Food Commission, 102 Gloucester Place, London WC1. Tel 071-935 9078.

Food Sense, (for publications from MAFF Food Safety Directorate), London SE99 7TT. Tel 081-694 8862.

Freedom Food Ltd, The Manor House, Causeway, Horsham, West Sussex RH12 1HG. Tel 0403 264181

Health Education Authority, Hamilton House, Mabledon Place, London WC1H 9TX. Tel 071-387 9528.

Ileostomy Association of Great Britain and Ireland, Amblehurst House, Chobham, Woking, Surrey GU24 8PZ.

Listeria Support Group, c/o Mark Horvath, Worlingwortth, Woodbridge, Suffolk IP13 7NZ.

Liver Support Group, Academic Department of Medicine, 10th Floor, Royal Free Hospital, London NW3 2QG.

The Soil Association, 86 Colston Street, Bristol BS1 5BB. Tel 0272 290661.

The Stroke Association, CHSA House, 123-127 Whitecross Street, London EC1Y 8JJ. Tel 071-490 7999.

The Vegan Society, 7 Battle Road, St Leonards-on-Sea, East Sussex TN37 7AA.

The Vegetarian Society, Parkdale, Dunham Road, Altrincham, Cheshire WA14 4QG.

Index